Health Secrets
of the Stone Age

What we can learn from deep in prehistory
to become leaner, livelier and longer-lived

Philip J. Goscienski M.D.

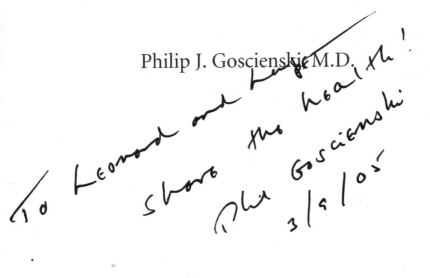

To Leonard and Longe the!
share the health!
Phil Goscienski
3/9/05

Health Secrets of the Stone Age

For information, permissions, or orders, contact

Philip J. Goscienski, M.D.
4938 Lassen Drive
Oceanside CA 92056
(760) 732-1414
Fax (760) 732-1499
drphilg@cox.net

The following publishers have generously given permission to quote from copyrighted works.

Page 167: from *The Prophet* by Kahlil Gibran, copyright 1923 by Kahlil Gibran and renewed 1951 by Administrators C.T.A. of Kahlil Gibran Estate and Mary G. Gibran. Used by permission of Alfred A. Knopf, a division of Random House, Inc.

Library of Congress Control Number: 2004095727
ISBN 0-9759102-0-5

Printed in the United States of America

Contents

Acknowledgements

C**OUNTLESS SCIENTISTS CONTRIBUTED** to the material that I have presented in this book, and their insight has helped me to form my own opinions. To them goes most of the credit for what you are about to explore within these pages. My special thanks go to Dr. S. Boyd Eaton, Dr. Marjorie Shostak and Dr. Melvin Konner, who wrote the *Paleolithic Prescription*. Their lucid explanations crystallized the hazy thoughts on this subject that had floated through my mind for a couple of decades.

It was my good fortune that I had excellent advice and continued support from so many friends and colleagues. In the earliest days, when the manuscript was only a collection of notes and outlines, Leigh Fenly, Children's Book Editor of the *San Diego Union-Tribune*, was an enthusiastic advisor, critic and coach. Roger Domingo and Dori O'Rourke, who had also overcome the obstacles that most authors face, were among my most enthusiastic supporters. Helpful comments came from neonatologist Dr. Nancy Wight, who gave me new insights regarding breastfeeding. Ted Walters, Dr. Chester Zelasko and Pat Zifferblatt of the Better Life Institute were generous in their encouragement. Dr. Sam Rehnborg and Dr. Aaron Crawford carefully reviewed the entire manuscript and verified concepts of which I was still unsure. Jacqueline Landis provided valuable help in editing the manuscript. Penny Sansevieri provided her expertise in publicity, and Robert Goodman designed the interior of the book. Leeza Hernandez transformed vague ideas into an eye-catching cover. Ellen Lohman's keen proofreader's eye caught the errors that had slipped past the rest of us.

Tom Hobbs posed for Stephanie Sundell of Creative Photography. Scott Mullins provided the artwork.

I am especially thankful for Pat, my loving, encouraging and patient wife of four and a half decades. Our children, Cathy, Chris, Elizabeth, Steve and Tom were gentle critics and ardent fans during a journey that was always illuminating, constantly challenging but never discouraging.

Finally, there was always the memory of our son, Michael, scholar, teacher, financier, advisor to government ministers, linguist and world traveler, who was with us for less than four decades but whose accomplishments and impact on the world of economics will outlive the rest of us, and to whom I dedicate this book.

Introduction

The first wealth is health.
– Ralph Waldo Emerson

Who would have predicted, at the beginning of the twentieth century, that health and fitness would have become a major industry before the beginning of the twenty-first? But what paradoxes we have before us! Walkers and joggers jostle through our parks, but the average American is heavier than ever. Experts tell us that we can avoid more than 80 percent of cancers, yet that disease remains near the top of the list of causes of death in the United States. The venerable pharmaceutical industry continues to grow, even as more than half the population admits to using alternative therapies. And in an age when knowledge of health and disease doubles every few years, the cost of medical care threatens to bankrupt our economy.

During a medical career that has spanned 4 decades I have puzzled over the blissful ignorance that most people, including physicians, have regarding the facts of living. I have watched our dearest friends' and relatives' health deteriorate, their lives shortened, as they suffer strokes and heart attacks and diabetes and the inability to enjoy their lives. On the other hand, I've known some people who are well into their 80s, who ski and scuba dive. I have watched them prance around castles in Europe and climb ancient Mayan ruins and flit through airports like adolescents. And I wondered why. Why the difference? Do they have secret knowledge?

There are secrets, but not in the sense of privileged and guarded information. They are principles that are apparent to anyone who has been keeping up, however modestly, with the enormous amount of health-related information pouring from our universities, medical schools and clinics. Like the craftsmen who patiently pick away at a modern work of art and find an old master underneath it, medical scientists are exposing health principles that our Stone Age ancestors practiced instinctively and unknowingly. Their studies affirm the transparent secret that your food style and your activity style will have a more profound effect on the way you look and feel, on your life span and your health span, than your genetic makeup or anything the science of medicine has to offer.

Getting older is what nature does to us; aging is what we do to ourselves. For centuries, humans have assumed that our physical abilities decline as we age. That is only true in late, late middle age. There is a slight decline in our ability to use oxygen as we add more years, and it's obvious that our skin becomes drier and our near vision changes. But muscle strength and speed diminish only slightly, unless we let them.

Did you know that in 1987 a 42-year-old won the Women's New York Marathon? In 1985 a 57-year-old placed second in the Mr. Olympia contest. There is an 1,100-mile dogsled race from Anchorage, Alaska to Nome, about the same as the distance between San Diego and Denver. Several years ago Norman Vaughan, 81 years old, came in fifth. Teiichi Igarashi climbed 12,300-foot Mount Fuji when he was 99 years old.

These are examples of vibrant living and successful aging, the goals that I would like all readers of this book to attain. The objective is not to live as long as possible, but to maintain optimal health as long as possible. In his poem *The Deacon's Masterpiece: The Wonderful One-Hoss Shay,* Oliver Wendell Holmes writes of a long and peaceful life that ends quickly and painlessly. The lives of Stone-Agers most often ended quickly, but seldom painlessly. Although our lives are longer, most of us pass through what Drs. Evans and Rosenberg, in *Biomarkers,* refer to as the Disability Zone. This is the period when we become increasingly dependent on others. The inevitable decline from good health to death should be a short one. For a disappointingly large segment of our population, that decline lasts for decades, the final years chairbound, dependent, financially drained, and anxious for release.

The pathfinders

Of the thousands of persons whose paths cross ours, only a handful will leave more than a shadowy imprint on our lives. The same is true of books. *The Paleolithic Prescription,* written by Eaton, Shostak and Konner, shed light on matters that had intrigued me since my middle years in medical school. Their *Discordance Hypothesis* succinctly explains why the so-called diseases of aging have suddenly, i.e., within the last three-quarters of a century, appeared to be so widespread in the most affluent societies, but not in the poorer ones.

The late, renowned cardiologist, Paul Dudley White, observed that in his earliest years of practice, myocardial infarction (heart attack) was an extremely uncommon cause of death. Last year it took the life of almost one-half million Americans. The story of type 2 diabetes is similar. No physician specialized in diabetes at the beginning of the last century, for it was not a common disease. Today's diabetologists proclaim that we are experiencing an epidemic of this disease among adults, and fear that the epidemic is spreading to children. In *The Paleolithic Prescription,* Eaton and his colleagues have made a detailed, anthropologist's analysis of prehistoric as well as contemporary hunter-gatherer lifestyles, in several areas of the globe, to explain these and other disease patterns.

This book — a different perspective

In Chapter One I will show how closely we resemble our distant ancestors, and why our disease patterns differ from theirs. The answer is not, as most people immediately rush to tell me, because they didn't live long enough to develop chronic diseases.

Our evolutionary origins tell us why diets fail, why calories sometimes matter and sometimes don't, why men lose weight more easily than their mates, and why Nature intended for your child to be a picky eater. The chapters on food and nutritional supplements will help you to make healthy choices without a calculator, without confusion, and without guilt. They will also help you to save many times as much money as the price of this book.

As you scan the Table of Contents you won't find a chapter on recipes. You don't need new menus, unfamiliar foods or exotic additions to gain health or to lose weight. Appendix 4 lists some books that together offer hundreds of healthy recipes for those who are looking for a change. For readers who worry that the Stone Age theme of this book includes raw meat, no meat or all meat, be assured that it does not. There is no need for a rigid foodstyle. Where I do make dietary recommendations, you'll find that they are not dull, difficult, demanding or discouraging.

Finally, this book is based on authoritative, well-researched and very recent information. Where there are areas of significant disagreement or inconclusive studies, I have tried to point them out. I also realize, however, that sometimes yesterday's certainty is today's doubt and tomorrow's error. I do not believe that truth is relative. It is simply elusive.

One

Your body is older than you are

HOW OLD ARE you? Not your body, but your genes. That answer is the key to understanding why we get tired, why we get fat, why we get sick and why we get old. It was during the Old Stone Age, which began some 3 million years ago, that our body chemistry nearly reached its current stage of development. The most important premise of this book is simple: the way our bodies function is virtually unchanged from those who lived hundreds of thousands of years ago but our lifestyle is vastly different. Since the Agricultural Revolution began about 12,000 years ago, the discordance between our genetic blueprint and our lifestyle has accelerated. The result is a biological disaster. This forms the Discordance Hypothesis of Drs. Eaton, Konner and Shostak, authors of *The Paleolithic Prescription*.

Obesity and type 2 diabetes do not occur in primitive populations or in wild animals; both disorders are extremely common in the United States and each is increasing by several percent every decade. At the beginning of the twentieth century myocardial infarction (heart attack) was almost a medical curiosity. It now causes almost a half-million deaths per year. Stroke is the third leading cause of death in the United States. The National Cancer Institute tells us that we can avoid 80 percent of cancers by changing our lifestyle.

Life was short for those who lived during the Stone Age because of diseases that modern medicine, with a strong assist from modern plumbing, has almost totally eliminated. However, their nutritional health was excellent. The health challenges that we encounter now are almost entirely of our own doing. We will find the remedies to these challenges in the Stone Age, whose "secrets" are uncovered in the pages that follow.

Introducing Sam and Sal

SAM and SAL are acronyms for Stone Age Man and Stone Age Lady. They represent our prehistoric ancestors and it is important to recognize that their bodies were almost identical to ours in every way. Evolution is a very slow process and we can show this by comparing ourselves, strictly in biological terms, with chimpanzees. The external differences between humans and chimps are obvious, even at some distance. But our eyes work the same way, and so do our kidneys, our intestines and reproductive organs, with minor differences. In terms of what is called genetic distance, only 1.6 percent of genes separate us from chimpanzees. As an example, Hemoglobin A, the main component of the oxygen-carrying chemical in our blood cells, has 297 amino acids. The number and type are identical in chimpanzee Hemoglobin A.

How do we explain this closeness in our genes and our very obvious differences in outward appearance? Genetic anthropologists may have the answer. Among the primate groups, including humans, molecular evolution has slowed down as morphologic evolution has speeded up. In other words, very small changes in the genes that are responsible for our outward appearance seem to produce what appear to us as large changes in body shape and facial features. To a nonbiologist there is a striking difference between the body size, skin color and facial characteristics of a tall Norwegian and a small Indonesian. From a biologist's point of view, these are really not large changes, for these persons are virtually identical in every aspect of their body chemistry, including blood types, digestive enzymes and immune systems.

Consider then how close our biological proximity is to our Stone Age ancestors, whose genetic distance from us must be very small. If we could go back 50,000 years and stand side by side with Sam and Sal, all of us dressed alike and with similar hair styles, no one who passed by could be sure which were the modern ones, although it's certain that our ancestors would be more muscular and probably taller. A few blood tests wouldn't show much of a difference either, except that you and I would probably have a blood cholesterol level nearly 100 milligrams higher than Sam or Sal's. We could go back much further, perhaps a half-million years, and find that those very ancient ancestors would not draw attention if they were to stroll through a shopping plaza dressed in modern clothing.

Because of the extremely high risk of death due to trauma and infection fifty millennia ago, barely 1 in 10 humans reached age 60. It would be a challenge to find elderly versions of Sam and Sal. If we did, they would still be muscular and agile, with little body fat, normal blood pressure and strong, dense bones. When death came it would not be due to a heart attack or stroke, or diabetes or cancer. Those are modern maladies, not ancient ones. Things over which he had no control killed Sam: injury, infection and predators — both animal and human. In contrast, most modern humans kill themselves, not by outright suicide but by the lifestyle they choose: poor diet, little exercise, alcohol and tobacco. These four factors, all of which are entirely within our ability to manage, account for more than 80 percent of mortality in the United States (Centers for Disease Control, Deaths, Preliminary Data for 2002).

How do we know that Sam and Sal were so robust, and that those who survived to a relatively old age were so healthy by our standards? Let us go to the fossil record of the Stone Age. We'll use that term

**The ten leading causes of death
in the United States, 2002**

Diseases of the heart
Cancer
Cerebrovascular disease (stroke)
Chronic lower respiratory diseases
Accidents
Diabetes mellitus
Influenza and pneumonia
Alzheimer's disease
Kidney disease

instead of Paleolithic or Neolithic. Paleolithic simply means *old stone age* and covers the millennia during which man developed primitive stone, bone and flint tools and wandered in small bands as he hunted and gathered for subsistence. During the Neolithic period (*new stone age*) man developed more sophisticated tools, pottery, weaving, and the earliest forms of agriculture and animal husbandry. The Stone Age was the period of human existence before writing but not before language. It was the time when people lived in small groups but not yet in villages or towns. Every person or family gathered their own food every day, whether animal or vegetable, and food storage by humans was about as sophisticated as that of squirrels. And it was a time when 99.9 percent of our genetic makeup had already been established.

Most people believe that our remote, i.e., Stone Age, ancestors had a hard life, were often undernourished, were not very robust and frequently faced famine. It is certainly true that they had a hard life. In spite of that, Stone Agers were muscular and strong, and human bones of the period are thick-walled and broad. Those areas of skeletal bone where muscles were attached are as prominent as those of today's best athletes. In the Mediterranean basin, 30,000-year-old skeletons indicate that the average height for males was about 5 feet 9.75 inches. Some skeletons discovered by the Leakey-Walker group reached a height of 6 feet 2 inches. It is only in the past century that the average person in affluent Western societies has become that tall. Even today, in Greece and Turkey, the average height for men and women has not yet reached that of hunter-gatherers from that region of 40,000 years ago.

In the hundreds of thousands of years when animals were abundant and people were not, in areas and at times not affected by ice ages, food was plentiful. Consider that when the early explorers of North America wrote of game, they described herds of buffalo that took days to pass, and enormous flocks of birds that darkened the skies. Serious famine was unlikely in the Stone Age for several reasons. Sam and Sal had an abundantly varied diet that included

> ### A misperception
>
> *A frequently asked question: Didn't Stone Agers die too early to get heart disease and stroke? The vast majority of them did; most died in infancy, usually from infectious diseases. The strength of our argument rests with observations on modern hunter-gatherers, who live the Stone Age lifestyle, suffer from similar infections, and do not have access to modern medical care. Many of them reach the sixth or seventh decade of life without the chronic diseases of civilization.*

hundreds of types of vegetation in the temperate and tropical areas in which they lived. Plant blights and insects have a limited range of hosts so that more species would be spared than would be affected by disease or pests. Many wild plants are drought-resistant, having developed that characteristic during eons of cyclical prolonged dry spells. Sam had a wide choice of small game. As weapon-making and hunting skills advanced, he had access to enormous numbers of large animals. He and the other members of his band could also rely on insects, grubs and worms, and these were probably not just a last resort if other sources dwindled.

We can gain some insight into the health of our ancestors by investigating the modern hunter-gatherer, the present-day equivalent of Sam and Sal. About 100 such groups exist on earth today, virtually all of them living in marginally sufficient environments, driven there by modern conquistadors. In spite of that, when we examine their health status and review causes of death, some conditions that modern physicians are familiar with are missing.

They are not obese. They do not have hypertension. Adult-onset diabetes is absent, and so is osteoporosis. Cancer is rare. These are not statistical aberrations in a society whose members die so quickly that such conditions don't have time to occur. At autopsy, Western young adult accident victims already have obvious arteriosclerotic changes in the major blood vessels. Young hunter-gatherers do not. Trowell and Burkitt described the findings of Drury in autopsies of 400 Ugandans over the age of 60 conducted at the Makerere University Medical School. There were only three deaths due to coronary heart disease (less than 1 percent); among African-Americans in the United States the rate is several times as high. Only nine died of hypertension. That disorder is almost epidemic now among African-Americans.

Even Drury's East African patients were somewhat westernized. It is increasingly difficult to find and study population groups that have maintained diet and activity patterns similar to "pre-contact" hunter-gatherers. Eaton, Shostak and Konner described several such groups from various parts of the world in their book, *The Paleolithic Prescription.* All these groups share certain traits. They tend to be lean, with normal blood pressure and cholesterol, rarely have diabetes and have almost no heart disease of the type found in Western societies. A comparison of Inuit natives living a modern lifestyle and Siberian villagers in a traditional environment shows that the former are more likely to be obese and that high blood pressure corresponds with obesity. At the beginning of the twentieth century diabetes was almost nonexistent among Native Americans. Less than 100 years later the incidence was 45 percent among adults in some tribes.

In Hawaii, Dr. John McDougall made similar observations. As a medical practitioner among agricultural workers and their families, he dealt with a homogeneous population group, most of whom had a fairly similar lifestyle. He observed that the Japanese who first came to Hawaii and maintained their ancestral ways were healthy and vigorous into their old age. Their children and grandchildren, who abandoned the food habits of their immigrant forebears, were diabetic, with coronary artery disease and colon cancer. Women of that racial group, who eat a traditional Japanese diet, have the lowest rate of breast cancer in the world, but when they adopt an American-style diet the risk of breast cancer rises significantly.

The Agricultural Revolution: a mixed blessing

The Agricultural Revolution did not consist of a single explosive phenomenon that quickly and simultaneously engulfed all of humankind. It began in several different areas after the last great ice age, roughly twelve thousand years ago. Several millennia passed before most humans stopped living in isolated bands of twenty or thirty individuals and established fixed communities, or villages. Domestication of wild grains and animals meant that fewer individuals were needed to provide food so that others could specialize in crafts, soldiery, art and administration. Advances in the technology of food production have left 99 percent of us in first-world countries able to do something else with our lives. Food production and food preparation take almost no time at all, because in the United States, someone outside the home prepares 40 percent of our meals and we enjoy them as "dine-out" or "take-out." Today's homemaker spends a fraction of the time it took her mother or grandmother to prepare a meal.

Surely this has made every aspect of feeding our families and us better.

Or has it?

The Agricultural Revolution made it possible for man's intellect and creativity to soar. By the dawn of the Bronze Age he had built palaces and pyramids. As it gave way to the Iron Age he produced epic poetry, beautiful artworks, a system of philosophy and complex legal codes. But in the background were new infectious diseases, higher infant mortality, reduction in stature, iron deficiency and bone disorders. Almost half of our Stone Age ancestors died violently, but they did not suffer from epidemic infections, and fossil remains show no evidence of chronic or severe nutritional or disease stress. Rates of infectious diseases rose considerably almost everywhere after the Agricultural Revolution, due to the combination of increasing population density, the proximity of domesticated animals and poor nutrition.

The Agricultural Revolution gave us a more plentiful food supply, but not a more reliable and healthier one. It did just the opposite. Sam and Sal had dozens of fruits, roots, nuts and berries from which to choose. Early agriculturalists concentrated on a handful of crops, primarily grains, because they could cultivate them more easily. However, an unseasonable freeze or prolonged drought might wipe out a domestic crop; among wild plants, some will survive all but the most extreme climatic events.

From the earliest days of farming even to the present, poor management has led to crop failure, plant diseases, soil erosion and lowered nutritive value. Domestication of cereal grains led to a decrease in quality because of soil exhaustion. Harlan found that wild grains of Turkey have twice as much protein as domesticated grain grown in the same general area. Einkorn (wild) wheat has 50 percent more protein than hard red winter wheat, which is the most common type grown in the United States. The new farmers and their families paid a high price for the convenience of civilization. Their foods were deficient in most nutrients, so that smaller stature, chronic anemia, poor dental health and a shorter lifespan became the norm.

Consider the difference between wild and cultivated plants. Wild forms develop for a reproductive advantage, so they have abundant seeds and thick rinds, husks or shells. They have less starch and low sugar, more protein and fiber and about 50 percent more calcium. Cultivation of plants minimizes the reproductive advantage so that we can enjoy seedless grapes, grapefruit and watermelon. Modern shoppers want sweet, tender, juicy produce without blemishes and with thin external coverings for ease of preparation and enjoyment.

Agriculture has become chemically dependent on fertilizers, pesticides and preservatives. These additives produce higher yields at a lower cost but do not necessarily result in better nutrition. There is no question that they are contributing to environmental and health problems. Irrigation raises soil salinity and adversely affects yield and quality.

The domestication of animals for food probably originated at about the same time as the domestication of plants. The earliest farmers recognized that some of their crop could be used for feed and that it was easier to raise animals than to hunt them. Unfortunately this proximity to animals led to some of the most serious infectious diseases of mankind, such as smallpox, measles and tuberculosis, among others. From a nutritional point of view it produced the same kinds of problems as the domestication of grains: less diversity, greater susceptibility to disease and lowered nutritional value.

Sam hunted dozens of species of game, both large and small. Today's supermarket has only three types of large game: cattle, pigs and (young) sheep. Not that we would want some of Sal's favorites, such as mammoth, goat, horse, (adult) sheep, camel and buffalo. We probably wouldn't care for most of his small game, either. It included rodents and reptiles, not just rabbits and birds. Our small game is even more limited than our choices of large game: it consists almost entirely of turkey and chicken.

There were no epidemics in the Stone Age. People were simply too widely dispersed for infectious diseases to spread from band to band. The Agricultural Revolution made possible the aggregation of people in towns and cities, and for the first time in human history, epidemic diseases appeared. Plagues of various kinds decimated whole towns, cities and armies even before biblical writers described them. When our ancestors settled near water, malaria became epidemic. Soil and streams became fouled with filth, and parasites proliferated: amebiasis, hookworm and dysentery of various kinds now had a dense, stationary population of human hosts.

A crowded community of domesticated animals is just as susceptible as a human one. The lack of genetic diversity of an animal population that is massed in a small area means that a single microbial strain can infect it and possibly eliminate it in a short time. If the bacterium or virus doesn't do the job, drastic control measures will. The smoky columns from pyres of burning carcasses throughout England will remain long in the memory of everyone, even those outside that country, during the foot-and-mouth outbreak in the United Kingdom at the start of 2001.

The progressive lack of biodiversity among domestic plants and animals has reached an alarming level, according to the United Nations Food and Agriculture Organization. About 5 percent of breeds of farm animals have died out since the mid-1980s, taking with them genes that allowed them to resist disease and drought. From distant prehistory through 15 millennia since the start of the Agricultural Revolution, Homo sapiens has taken nourishment from some 10,000 plant species. Now more than 90 percent of his food supply comes from only 17 cultivated species.

Animals in the wild have a more diverse diet than those raised in pens, so their nutritional value is higher. Just as Sam and Sal had an abundance of plants from which to choose, so did the creatures they hunted. Wild animals eat a variety of grasses and plants, with seasonal differences, growing in soil that has not been repeatedly cultivated for the preceding hundreds of years. They are likely to ingest a wide array of minerals and micronutrients, including hundreds of phytonutrients. Domesticated animals generally are fed a limited number of foods, usually grains, which themselves are grown in nutrient-poor soil to which chemical fertilizers have been added. Those who dislike venison complain of its gamy flavor; hunters boast of its richness. The diversity of diet that changes the flavor of venison affects its food value, as well. Venison has twice as much iron as eye round of beef and four times as much as pork tenderloin. It has more niacin and riboflavin than beef.

Meat from wild game not only has less fat than that which comes from domesticated stock, but the quality is better suited to human nutrition. The omega-3 fatty acids have critical roles in the nourishment of the human brain and nervous system. Wild game has five times as much polyunsaturated fat with a high content of EPA (eicosa-pentaenoic acid), one of the important omega-3 fatty acids. Modern beef has almost undetectable levels of EPA.

> **Phytonutrients**
>
> *Phytonutrients are plant substances, numbering in the thousands that contribute to the well-being of the plants that produce them and the animals that eat the plants. Many are antioxidants, some act like hormones, and others block the action of cancer-producing substances.*

Farmers breed domestic animals for rapid weight gain, increased fat content, greater milk production and larger and more frequent offspring. In order to achieve these goals producers must confine the animals, restrict the diversity of their diet, castrate them and feed them antibiotics and hormones. These methods are very successful: domesticated animals have six times as much total fat and ten times as much saturated fat as animals in the wild.

During the Stone Age there was probably a wide range of meat intake from one group to another, but Sam and Sal and their contemporaries never had prime beef, or its equivalent, which has 38 percent fat. Wild game averages about 7 percent fat, or less. Medical authorities consider animal fat to be one of the major causes of arteriosclerosis and its complications of heart disease and stroke. But just as consumers prefer sweet and juicy fruit to that which has less sugar and more fiber, they prefer meat with the most fat. This preference for sweets and fats is universal, and it is one of the Secrets of the Stone Age.

Why do we prefer sweets and fats?

"Feast or famine" is a trite expression that observers use to describe business cycles. It has a more profound meaning in the context of health and nutrition. Extended famine was probably rare during the Stone Age, but periods of prolonged fasting or food scarcity were not. Migration, the end of the hunting season, a long winter or drought resulted in a diminished food supply. The evolutionary acquisition of the ability to store fat during times of abundance helped to guarantee survival. The fat we accumulate beneath our skin and around our internal organs is metabolically fairly inactive. In other words, it doesn't require much energy for upkeep, and is an excellent way to store calories for future use. A few hundred thousand years ago there was no knowledge of salting, smoking or drying. Even after our forebears developed these methods, it was still easier to carry stored energy as body fat than to keep it at the back of the cave or other shelter where it could be eaten by vermin or larger animals. Although sweets as we know them were rarely available to Sam and Sal, we all have an appetite for them, as well as for fat. That's because we can convert most forms of sugar to fat very efficiently. Hundreds of thousands of years ago this was an advantage. In times of abundance, an appetite for fat becomes helpful in future survival. Evolution has left us all with "fat genes," which allow us to accumulate body fat so that we can survive the next food shortage. In the past few generations, developed societies have eliminated food shortages or famines. Feasting is now unopposed by food scarcity, and its consequences are the leading causes of death in developed countries.

A person is usually considered to be obese if his or her body weight is 20 percent more than the standard for that population. For the average person that is about 30 pounds over standard weight. Body Mass Index measurement (Chapter Three) is becoming the current norm. Obesity is not a twentieth-century phenomenon, but it has been accelerating dramatically in only the past few decades. In 1971, 1 in 8 Americans was obese; in 2001 it was 1 in 4. Sixty-four percent of us are overweight, and that number is expected to rise to 70 percent before the end of this decade. When Yankee stadium was rebuilt after about 70 years the seats had to be made 2 inches wider to accommodate the more generous posteriors of the fans. The nation's largest casket company reports that sales of oversize caskets increased by 20 percent between 1996 and 2001.

Dozens of genes determine fat uptake and distribution. In spite of the common perception that we are not in control of our body weight because we have the wrong genetic makeup, all these genes have been present in humans for tens of thousands, perhaps hundreds of thousands, of years. But only in the past century has obesity been so common. Heredity is not predestination, and the story of the Pima Indians clearly proves that point.

About 800 years ago the Pima Indians of the American southwest split into two groups. One group settled in the area that is now southern Arizona. The other group moved into the Sierra Madre Mountains of Mexico. By the 1970s most of the Indians of Arizona were no longer farming. They were living the American lifestyle, with 40 percent of their calories coming from fat. That group of Indians, according to Dr. Eric Ravussin of the National Institutes of Diabetes and Kidney Diseases, has the highest incidence of obesity reported for any population group in the entire world. They also have the highest incidence of type 2 diabetes that has ever been recorded.

The genetic makeup of this Native American population includes the so-called thrifty gene. It allows them to store fat rapidly when food is abundant. As a survival factor, the thrifty gene enables them to make it through periods of deprivation, clearly an advantage for those whose food supply is not predictable at every season.

What happened to the Pima Indians who went to Mexico, and who also have the thrifty gene? They still ranch and farm, and spend more than 40 hours a week doing physical labor. Their diet contains 20 percent fat instead of 40 percent. Their average weight is 57 pounds less than their relatives in Arizona. They are about 1 inch shorter. Very few of them have diabetes. Hypertension, coronary artery disease and stroke are rare, and they are robust in their old age.

Some scientists frankly consider obesity an epidemic, and the reasons, more evident in the United States than in most countries, are very obvious. No matter what one's genetic makeup happens to be, gaining weight is a matter of taking in more calories than one uses.

Food pyramids

In 1992 the USDA published the Food Guide Pyramid, a diagram that indicates the types and quantities of foods that comprise a healthy diet. The base of the pyramid (Fig. 1, page 25) is made up of grains (bread, cereal, rice, pasta). Where did Sam and Sal get these foods? The answer is that they did not. Grain production did not exist until about 12,000 years ago, and the wild grains that earlier people consumed must have been a very small part of their diet. Wheat is hardly a convenience food. Gathering wheat requires cutting tools, and after threshing and separation of the grains, the

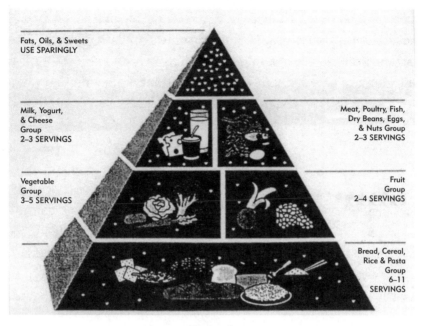

Fats, Oils, & Sweets
USE SPARINGLY

Milk, Yogurt,
& Cheese
Group
2–3 SERVINGS

Meat, Poultry, Fish,
Dry Beans, Eggs,
& Nuts Group
2–3 SERVINGS

Vegetable
Group
3–5 SERVINGS

Fruit
Group
2–4 SERVINGS

Bread, Cereal,
Rice & Pasta
Group
6–11
SERVINGS

Figure 1

edible portion must be separated from the husk. This is hardly easy and requires both heat and mechanical grinding.

Nowhere is the discordance between our body chemistry and food intake more obvious than in this dependence on grain-based foods. When cereal grains almost completely replaced fruits, vegetables and animal protein, the average person's stature diminished by several inches and his lifespan by several years. Infant mortality climbed. Bone and tooth disorders increased, and so did infectious diseases and iron-deficiency anemia.

The USDA recommends 2 to 3 servings of milk, yogurt and cheese among the 15 to 21 total food servings. The only milk available in the Stone Age came from lactating human females, and none was available after the first 2 to 4 years of life. Cheese, yogurt and other milk products did not come into existence until the Agricultural Revolution. A significant number of people, especially non-Caucasians, do not tolerate dairy products well. The digestive enzyme lactase, which helps us digest lactose, or milk sugar, begins to decline in most people, and in some population groups it is absent after the age of about 6 years in roughly 80 percent. This is an example of *bioeconomics*, the evolutionary phenomenon that discards a metabolic process that is no longer useful to the organism.

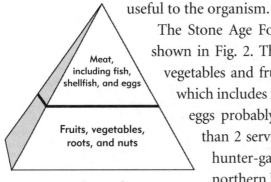

The Stone Age Food Guide Pyramid is shown in Fig. 2. The base is made up of vegetables and fruits. The second level, which includes meat, poultry, fish and eggs probably accounted for more than 2 servings. In some modern hunter-gatherer groups of northern latitudes meat and fish alone form almost the entire pyramid, for there are no local grains or fruits, and vegetables are rare. The tip of the USDA pyramid contains fats, oils and sweets, but these were also almost nonexistent tens of thousands of years ago. Wild game has little fat. The production of vegetable oils requires presses. The only sweet was honey, and that was not always available.

Figure 2

The Stone Age Food Guide Pyramid seems to indicate that meat comprised a sizeable portion of their diet. That was probably true for the late Stone Age, perhaps 50,000 or 100,000 years ago, when humans developed effective hunting weapons. Before that period, extending about 2 million years to the precursors of Homo sapiens, vegetarianism predominated. When they developed the bow and arrow about 20,000 years ago, humans became so efficient at hunting that several large species became extinct. After that time overhunting reduced big game animals, and the proportion of meat in the diet fell. It dropped again after the start of the Agricultural Revolution when societies became grain-based.

The most striking difference between the wild game eaten by Sam and Sal and the supermarket product of today is the fat content, as noted in Table 1, below.

Wild game	Grams of fat/ 100 grams	Modern meats	Grams of fat/ 100 grams
rabbit	3.5–5.0	chicken breast	7.6–8.7
moose	1.0–1.5	turkey, light	8.3
pheasant	5.2	veal	13.1
elk	1.9	ground beef	20.9–21.2
bison	2.4–3.0	lamb (loin)	23.1–32.0
deer	3.2–4.0	ham	18.5–29.1
		sirloin steak	16.7–26.7

Table 1

According to the USDA Food Guide Pyramid we should use fats, sweets and oils sparingly. But sparingly doesn't sell, either in the supermarket or in restaurants. Fats add texture and flavor to baked goods. There are some very acceptable substitutes for the home chef and I have listed these in Chapter Six, but commercial recipes still rely on the cheaper and more convenient fats and oils.

The only sweetener available to Sam and Sal was honey. People living in the Mediterranean Basin grew sugar cane 2,000 years ago, but sugar was an expensive luxury until the nineteenth century. Since then, per capita intake of sugar has increased steadily, especially in the past century. The average American takes in more than one-third of a pound of sugar every day. That represents approximately 20 percent of the average daily caloric intake, several hundred calories that provide energy but no other food value.

Although alcohol is obviously not included in the food pyramid, it provides 7 to 10 percent of the average caloric intake in the United States. If that seems like a lot, consider that two glasses of wine, each about three and a half ounces, contain 200 to 300 calories. Two beers or two mixed drinks contain about the same number. Thus, almost one-third of the calories Americans take in on a daily basis come from sugar and alcohol, which contain no vitamins, no minerals, no trace elements and no fiber.

In various publications, Drs. S. Boyd Eaton, S. B. Eaton III, M. Konner and M. Shostak have drawn from scores of studies of ancient and modern hunter-gatherer societies. They show how during a tiny fraction of his existence, Homo sapiens has transformed himself from a creature perfectly aligned with his environment to one who has to exert an enormous amount of intellect and imagination to correct "the selected features of our current bioenvironmental milieu." In Table 2 I have adapted from their publications some of the major dietary differences between Stone Age and contemporary American cultures.

	Stone Age	Contemporary American
Dietary protein	33 percent	12 percent
Carbohydrate	46 percent	46 percent
Fat	21 percent	42 percent
Fiber	60–150 grams	10–20 grams
Sodium	700 milligrams	2,300-6,900* milligrams
Calcium	1,500–2,000 milligrams	740 milligrams
Sugar	rare	1/3 lb. / day
Vitamin C	440 milligrams	88 milligrams
Alcohol	none	7–10 % of daily calories

*This higher figure is reported from Japan.
N.B.: When Homo sapiens became a skilled hunter his protein intake rose significantly. Throughout most of his existence on earth his protein intake was more moderate.

Table 2

Work and exercise

The dietary discordance between ancient humans and modern ones is only one side of the issue. Activity patterns show the same discordance and may even be more important. Sam and Sal were muscular and lean because their lifestyle required much physical labor. It wasn't until late in the nineteenth century — well into the Industrial Revolution — that motor power replaced muscle power. Since the early 1900s, physical activity among Americans has declined by more than 75 percent.

How did our ancestors prior to the Industrial Revolution get their food? Most of them lived on farms, and milked cows by hand twice a day. They hoed their fields and walked behind a plow. They sowed seed by hand and threshed grain with sticks. Those who didn't farm had equally strenuous occupations. Miners used picks and shovels; lumbermen used axes and saws. Delivery people carried packages in their arms, or pulled carts, or drove wagons.

Household chores provided plenty of exercise until the mid-twentieth century. My mother and her generation used a washboard and turned a crank as they put clothes through a wringer. Laundry dried on a clothesline, not in a gas dryer. Taking it off the line wasn't much easier than putting it on, especially when it froze in the winter. The women who had to iron did it with appliances that weighed several times what they weigh now, and it took them longer. Anyone affluent enough to own a carpet had to beat the dust out with a carpet-beater. Until just a few score years ago, they had to carry water from a well.

Our forebears did these things well into their 60s and 70s. Twenty-first-century hunters and gatherers still do. The women of those societies often forage three or four miles away from their shelter, carrying back several pounds of fruits and berries and roots. Men cover a hunting range several miles in diameter and bring their quarry home on their backs.

The crude tools that Sam and Sal used to gather food, build shelters, make clothing and defend themselves required a huge output of energy. Tools in first-world countries are engine-driven, electrically powered and electronically steered. Even fingertip control is old technology; the few grams of muscle that control our voice-box will soon be all we need to direct the work processes that we have not already delegated to the computer.

It isn't necessary to adopt the lifestyle of the hunter-gatherer in order to take advantage of what nature has provided for us during the millions of years it took to become what we are today. Nor is it necessary to exercise several hours a day or to make severe changes in our dietary habits. In Chapter Two I'll describe the Seven Promises. In later chapters you will find out how these promises can be fulfilled within the context of the modern lifestyle.

Two

The seven promises

* *You will feel better*
* *You will look better*
* *You will be stronger*
* *You will be safer*
* *You will not be hungry*
* *You will not have to count calories*
* *You will save money*

THESE SEVEN PROMISES represent goals that no fad diet programs are able to deliver. If they could we would have only a handful of weight loss and fitness methods instead of hundreds. Book distributors could stock the works of just a few authors on the subject of health instead of more than a thousand. Yo-yo dieting would cease to exist and 60 percent of the United States population would not be overweight, as it is today. These promises become self-evident when you understand what the Stone Age lifestyle was like and how you can adopt its best elements. You will recognize these Seven Promises in the chapters that follow.

You will feel better

Fat weight is dead weight and the average American is carrying around about 30 pounds of it. It seems impossible that if you gain only about one-third of an ounce per week — about as much as a birthday card weighs — you will have gained about 30 pounds between your 25th and 55th birthdays. Yet, that's how this creeping obesity occurs, in tiny, unnoticeable increments. When you remove all or most of that burden in a few weeks or months by a change in eating habits and regular exercise, it's no surprise that you will have less fatigue, greater endurance and a general feeling of well being.

This book offers an eating plan, not a diet plan, although most overweight people who follow the suggestions I make will lose weight. Almost everyone will lose fat and gain muscle. If you need to lose some extra weight, this regimen will allow you to do it slowly, a pound or two per month. That probably seems too slow compared to the quickie diets touted on TV and posted on light poles around the country, but it's safe, healthy, and won't sap your energy. After all, you weren't aware of the weight when you put it on; you shouldn't be aware of it when you take it off.

There is another reason why removing fat from your body as well as from your table is going to make you feel better. I once saw a film, taken through a microscope, of blood flowing through the smallest blood vessels, or capillaries, of a rabbit's ear. The first frames showed blood cells racing through those tiny vessels. The next sequence was taken after the animal ate a high-fat meal, and the slowing of blood flow was so dramatic that it was almost like looking at a still photograph. This may explain why a diet high in saturated fat causes a decrease in performance on memory tasks and slows down the rate of learning in laboratory animals.

After a fatty meal, blood flow slows down because of the increased viscosity, or thickness, of the blood. This results in the inefficient delivery of oxygen and nutrients, which affects every organ, and may increase the risk of a heart attack. I dislike giving a lecture after lunch or dinner because I know that many people in that audience have had a high-fat meal and blood is flowing through their brains about as fast as it did through that rabbit's ear. Think about how you felt last Thanksgiving, after a typical 4,000-calorie meal (sidebar). Does it make sense that when your circulatory system is carrying the minimal amount of fat, giving you the maximal flow of blood and oxygen, you will feel better?

Calories in a typical Thanksgiving dinner	
3 handfuls salted mixed nuts (4 oz.)	*680*
5 crackers with cheese	*300*
2 servings turkey, 8 oz., no skin, lt/dk	*400*
1 scoop mashed potatoes (½ c.)	*110*
1 serving candied sweet potatoes	*200*
2-3 ladles gravy (3 oz.)	*300*
1½ helpings stuffing	*225*
cranberry sauce (1/4 c.)	*100*
creamed peas and pearl onions (½ c.)	*120*
1 serving green beans	*30*
2 rolls, 1 tbsp. butter	*300*
2 pieces apple pie (not a la mode)	*800*
1 12-oz. beer	*150*
1 glass red wine	*120*
2 oz. chocolate	*300*
2 cups coffee, half-and-half, 1 tsp sugar	*80*
Total calories	**4015**

Eating a large meal sometimes precedes a heart attack. There may be more than one reason, such as increased blood pressure following a heavy meal, or a rise in insulin, but it may be due to an increased likelihood of blood clot formation. When there is a rise in the blood level of certain fats, such as those found in animal products, there is a corresponding rise in a blood component that increases clot formation. It is the same component that initiates the formation of a clot inside a coronary artery and causes a heart attack. Even in healthy young men, a high-fat meal decreases blood flow in these critical vessels that provide oxygen to the heart.

Muscle is one of the storehouses of glycogen, also known as animal starch. (The other is the liver.) When the level of blood sugar (glucose) is greater than our immediate needs, we store it as glycogen until those reserves are full. The greater the muscle mass the more glycogen it can hold. Sam and Sal had a large muscle mass so that they could store more energy than most of us, but we have the same basic genetic endowment that they had. We just haven't nurtured it.

Looking good

Do you think that your body is shaped like Nature intended? I suggest that you take a look at the inside cover of Body for Life, by Bill Phillips (Harper Collins publ., 1999). You might not want to make that commitment to fitness, and you don't have to in order to have a very healthy lifestyle, but it will show you what ordinary humans can do.

The brain makes hormones called endorphins, which are natural pain-relievers and mood elevators. You can't buy endorphins in a bottle (yet). You have to make your own, and you can do this just by exercising. Exercise elevates mood in the long term as well as the short term. Those who exercise regularly have lower rates of depression.

Feeling better includes feeling better about yourself. It's hardly a secret that people who are overweight often have a poor self-image. That leads to a vicious cycle in which lower self-esteem leads to excess eating which, in turn, leads to more obesity, lower self-esteem, and so on. It's possible to reverse that cycle. Your overall appearance will improve when you have lost just a few pounds of fat, and so will your self-confidence. The moderate physical activity that I describe in Chapter Four will give you an added sense of well-being and accomplishment that will make it easier to continue to make improvements in your lifestyle. You will learn in the following pages that cravings are not a sign of weakness and that there are biological reasons that explain why it gets progressively harder to lose more weight. Insight will replace frustration.

Among our suggestions, and one that has had a most enthusiastic response in our seminar audiences, is that you should not weigh yourself every day, or every week, or every month. In fact, I suggest that you weigh yourself only two times a year: once on your birthday and once between birthdays. Daily weighing makes no sense at all and only contributes to anxiety and stress by reinforcing the feeling that you are making no progress. Your weight can fluctuate by a pound or more within hours, depending on food intake, bladder contents (the urine in a moderately full bladder can weigh half a pound), bowel evacuation and sweating. The goal is not to lose weight, but to lose fat. On most weight reduction regimens the early drop is water loss. Losing fat is a slow process and it sometimes provokes a sense of failure unless we understand the transformation we're making. Muscle weighs more than fat but takes up much less space. Someone who loses ten pounds of fat and replaces it with ten pounds of muscle will weigh the same, but will obviously look trimmer and feel better. Thus the scale doesn't reveal anything that the mirror won't, or that our clothing won't. Free yourself from the slavery of the scale and you will feel better.

You will look better

"You look wonderful! Have you lost weight?" Isn't that one of the most uplifting comments we can hear? Have you ever met an old friend who looked younger than his or her chronological age? What made them look younger? The answer might be plastic surgery, but more than likely it's because they are more slender than other friends of similar vintage.

People who look younger than their chronological age are usually the ones who have been able to avoid putting on the extra ounces that stealthily slither onto our frame starting at about the age of 25. Whether it's the upper arm or lower face, the more fat there is under the skin the more it will sag. Wrinkling is inevitable because our skin loses elasticity as we get older. The cherubic cheeks we had as three-year-olds are just following the law of gravity as they sink below our jaw line.

> **Smoke signals**
>
> *Those who smoke generally look older than those who do not. The skin of smokers contains larger amounts of an enzyme called metalloproteinase, which degrades collagen, one of the supporting elements of skin structure.*

When regular exercise adds muscle to our bodies it distributes itself as Nature intended. An excess accumulation of fat disturbs the body's architecture because most of it, especially in men, accumulates around the waist. When the abdomen enlarges the center of gravity moves forward. The lower spine curves inward and produces a swaybacked appearance. Your carriage and posture will improve as you increase your muscle mass and muscle tone and your waist becomes smaller. That may be all it takes to relieve back and knee pain, or even to eliminate the need for back surgery or knee replacement.

You will be stronger

Do you think that you can double your strength in 30 days? That's not just a likely estimate, it's a conservative one. Nursing-home patients in Boston were able to triple their strength in 8 weeks after starting a weight-training program. For persons at any age, being stronger means that games and athletic activities become easier and more fun. For the older individual, the sense of well-being that accompanies increased strength and vigor, and the lessened need to rely on others for help with the daily chores of life, are priceless.

Whether you're carrying groceries or grandchildren, you'll do it more easily when you're fit.

There's an enormous difference between weight lifting, an Olympic sport, and resistance exercise. The physical activity that I will describe in later chapters is meant for conditioning, not competition.

You will be safer

Prolonged bed rest, the weightlessness of space travel and lack of exercise all contribute to three things that increase the risk of injury: decreased strength, weaker bone structure and a diminished sense of balance.

Muscles get smaller as we age, but it's not the years that matter. Creeping obesity hides the subtle sabotage that we inflict upon ourselves when we avoid physical activity. As I'll explain in Chapter Four, bones get weaker for the same reason that muscles do.

Many medical conditions that are not under our control can affect our balance, including brain disorders and inner ear problems. The frequency of these is inconsequential compared to muscle wasting that results from inactivity, which is the single most important reason why elderly persons lose their balance and injure themselves in falls.

You will not be hungry

I have described meal strategies that are based on elements of the prehistoric lifestyle and that will keep you satisfied from hunger all day long. In Chapter Three I'll explain the difference between calorie-dense and calorie-sparse foods. Sam and Sal had access only to the latter. The calorie-sparse foods that formed the core of the human diet until the Agricultural Revolution included fruits, roots, nuts, and vegetables. Unlike modern produce, they contained much more fiber and were quite filling. Modern foods, with their high levels of sugar, white flour and fat, allow us to take in a large number of calories before we satisfy our appetite.

Our prehistoric ancestors didn't confine their eating to three times a day. They were grazers just like modern primates, and were not often hungry for very long. Hunger hinders our brain, saps our muscle strength, thins our temper and lowers our thresholds for anger and frustration. When we limit our meal patterning to three meals a day, or fewer, we experience hunger pangs and cravings. If our meal schedule is off by just an hour or two, cravings lead to stress and unwise choices of snacks. In Chapter Nine you will find how effortless it is to control hunger.

You will not have to count calories

Even if it were easy to count calories, the thought of doing it for the rest of your life is hardly motivating. But it isn't easy. When researchers tested knowledgeable and well-motivated people on their ability to estimate their calorie intake on a daily basis they found that almost no one was able to count them accurately. In fact, study subjects undercounted by approximately 20 percent. For a 2,500-calorie diet, that's 500 calories! And those people knew they were being monitored. It is also not necessary to meticulously calculate intake of fat, protein, carbohydrate or cholesterol. There are simple techniques for picking tasty foods, which are consistently low in fat and cholesterol, and avoiding those that are not. With the strategies outlined later you will make selections at the supermarket and restaurant effortlessly without the need of a calculator.

You will save money

Fat is expensive. So are sugar treats and alcohol. On the other hand, fat gives a meal its palatability and flavor, and sugar its pleasantness. Alcohol in moderation stimulates the appetite and may have some health benefits. I don't advocate eliminating fat, sugar or alcohol but I do promote modifying our use of all three in order to have better health and lower food costs. Investigators at the George Washington University Lipid Research Clinic studied two groups of families. One group averaged 37 percent fat in their diet — about what is normal for American families. The other families got only about 10 percent of their calories from fat. When the researchers analyzed each group's food costs they found that the low-fat family spent an average of $40 per week less than the typical family. That's a difference of about $2,000 per year.

How much will the average family of four save each month by NOT buying:		
1 qt. ice cream	$4.00 – 7.20/week	$16 – 29/month
1 cheesecake		$7.40 – 20.00/month
2 pies per month		$9.00 – 14.40/month
1 box chocolate chip cookies		$4.00/month
1 box Oreo cookies		$3.60/month
1 box oatmeal-raisin cookies		$3.35/month
1 box misc. cookies		$3.00/month
1 layer cake		$8.10/month
1 dozen donuts		$3.00/month
1 jar chocolate syrup		$2.80/month
	Total monthly savings	$60.25–94.25

You will see these Seven Promises fulfilled in just a week or two. Notice that "You will lose weight" is not among them, although most other programs prominently proclaim that seductive promise. You can lose a few pounds quickly on a sharply restricted diet that is usually uncomfortable and sometimes dangerous. However, an eating regimen that differs greatly from our normal pattern is virtually impossible to maintain for a lifetime. The fact that about 90 percent of dieters are back to — or above — their starting weight within five years is well known to researchers, and to most of the general public. No matter how much you want to lose weight, that is not a goal that will motivate you. On the other hand, the Seven Promises taken together form a constellation of reasonable, attainable, satisfying goals which are consistent with our deepest values: self-preservation, self-esteem and self-fulfillment.

Three

Body wisdom: why dieting is not meant to work

SAM AND SAL ate less only when there was less to eat. This might have occurred during migration, on an extended hunt, or near the end of an unusually prolonged and severe winter. The band in which they existed suffered no crop failures because they did not rely on a narrow range of foodstuffs. They could choose from scores of species of plants wherever they lived. Many of those plants had become resistant to drought and disease over many millennia, so some would always survive. Animal plagues that killed off some species of game would spare most others. There were no widespread human epidemics in the Stone Age because population density was too small to support them.

Did they fast deliberately? Perhaps the shamans of the late Stone Age did. When they discovered the mind-altering effects of intentional fasting they undoubtedly passed that lore on to their successors. But the deliberate avoidance of food is not a normal human behavior, and our earliest ancestors ate less than their bodies required only in times of scarcity. As I noted in Chapter One, the food supply was varied and fairly constant in the forests and savannahs of the African continent where Homo sapiens originated. That is not true in all parts of the populated world into which humans eventually

Overweight vs. obesity

In the past, overweight meant being a few pounds heavier than one's ideal weight as shown by a standard weight-for-height table. Obesity was a weight 20 percent greater than the standard table. Scientists now prefer Body Mass Index (BMI) and express it in kilograms per meter squared. To calculate your BMI, divide your weight in kilograms (pounds divided by 2.2) by the square of your height in meters (inches divided by 39.4). Overweight is defined as a BMI between 25.0 and 29.9 kg/m², obesity at 30.0 or more. You can determine your BMI in seconds at the web site www.caloriecontrol. org.

spread. In the lands that border the Pacific Ocean, for example, food deprivation occurred frequently enough so that over eons of evolutionary development, thrifty genes emerged, bestowing on some population groups the ability to store fat more easily during periods of plenty. That insured survival during periods of famine, and, though now unneeded, those protective traits persist. Among aboriginal peoples in Polynesia, Latin America and the Arctic, sudden Westernization has resulted in what responsible medical authorities call an epidemic of obesity and diabetes. For example, on the island state of Kosrae, in Micronesia, nearly 85 percent of inhabitants between the ages of 45 and 64 are obese and more than 25 percent are diabetic.

What happens when we starve ourselves

After the body has accumulated some fat, it releases it most grudgingly, as if anticipating a prolonged scarcity of energy. During a period of fasting, the metabolic rate ratchets downward in an attempt to match the decrease in energy intake. Persons who deliberately starve themselves by going on what we euphemistically refer to as a diet soon encounter the frustration of reaching a weight plateau in spite of taking in fewer calories. Unaware that they have set in motion a primitive survival mechanism, they may cut their caloric intake even more, yet see little further weight loss. Persons who do lose weight even under medical supervision may find that the last few pounds or inches are the hardest to lose. This is simply the body's ultimate attempt to prolong survival in the face of famine. In a calorie-restricted diet, the body gives up muscle as well as fat. Muscle burns a considerable number of calories, even at rest. When severe fasting diminishes some of that calorie-consuming muscle mass, the body requires less energy, and weight loss slows down.

Why do we lose muscle mass when we deprive ourselves of food? Probably because muscles are more expendable than other body parts. We can't restore our brain, heart and kidneys; we can rebuild muscle after a moderate fast (but not after frank starvation). In persons who lower their intake to 1,000 calories per day, and who do not exercise, the loss of lean body mass accounts for as much as 36 percent of the weight lost. Unfortunately, most dieters never replace that muscle.

Few dieters are aware that they can quickly deplete their vitamin stores, especially the B vitamins and vitamin C. When

> **Parents take note**
>
> *Dieting presents ominous implications for adolescents. Their risk of developing an eating disorder is several-fold higher than nondieters. Illness and growth failure are also more common in young persons who diet.*

they decrease food intake they also decrease the supply of minerals such as calcium. Without supplements, the woman who cuts her calories by 40 percent may lower her calcium intake by the same amount. If she loses muscle, the bone that supports that muscle will become less dense. Both factors contribute to the risk of osteoporosis.

Yo-yo dieting: the Sisyphus Syndrome

Those who go through cycles of weight gain and loss are referred to as yo-yo dieters. They have plenty of company. More than 90 percent of dieters regain most of their original weight within 2 to 5 years. Of those who lose more than 20 percent of their body weight, fewer than 5 percent will maintain that loss for more than 5 years. They do not realize that this is a biological success: their bodies are preparing for the next period of food scarcity.

> **Who was Sisyphus?**
>
> *Sisyphus was the mythological king of Corinth whose punishment for his greedy ways consisted of an eternity in Hades, pushing uphill a heavy stone that rolled back down again as soon as he reached the top.*

Sisyphus had it easy. He only had to roll the stone up the same hill every time. Yo-yo dieters (weight cyclers) have an additional challenge: their hill becomes progressively steeper. This is another natural adaptation for survival. When Sam and Sal lost weight because of a diminished food supply they regained it when their intake returned to normal. Individuals who go on fasting diets repeatedly are aware that it takes longer to lose the same amount of weight in each subsequent period of induced starvation. We cannot be certain that this occurred during prehistoric periods of food deprivation but the "Fat Rat" study suggests that possibility. When scientists placed a group of obese rats on a reduced-calorie diet, it took the animals 21 days to lose their excess weight. They regained it after they resumed their regular diet. When they returned to the same reduced-calorie intake as the first time, it took 46 days, more than two times as long, to lose the same amount of weight.

Several adverse effects accompany yo-yo dieting, not the smallest of which are the feelings of failure and low self-esteem that

> *Diet: a method of training the body to gain weight and to keep it on.*

result from repeated unsuccessful cycles of weight loss. There is some evidence that victims of this phenomenon have a higher rate of heart disease, although not all experts agree. The likelihood that yo-yo dieters start with a greater degree of obesity partly accounts for this increase, because obesity itself raises the risk of atherosclerosis, diabetes, hypertension and heart disease. Further, dieters often have poor fluid intake and become dehydrated. This may lead to poor oxygen supply to heart muscle and increases the chance of myocardial infarction (heart attack).

Yo-yo dieters and those who lose weight rapidly have an increased risk of gallbladder disease, especially women. Women are 2½ times as likely as men to have gallstones, probably because estrogen is responsible for an increase of cholesterol (the main component of gallstones) in bile. During pregnancy there is increased sludging of the gallbladder contents, and the gallbladder does not empty as efficiently after a meal. This may explain why the risk is higher in women who have had more pregnancies. Persons who lose weight rapidly have a 10-20 percent risk of developing gallstones, possibly because they are more likely to restrict their fluid intake. The risk is even higher in those who lose more than 3 pounds per week, or more than 24 percent of their initial body weight.

Not all physicians agree that weight cycling is harmful. Some weight cycling was inevitable for Sam and Sal, and our bodies are probably adapted to it in some degree. We are better equipped to handle occasional weight cycling than we are to carrying excessive fat stores for several decades.

How Americans diet and how they fail

What would Sam and Sal notice first if they strolled along a crowded beach today? The large number of obviously overweight persons would astound them. Obesity, even being overweight, was rare far back in prehistory. In the days when humans were part of the food chain and not at the top of it, obesity would have been a significant liability. Ancient artisans produced "Venus" figurines   that sometimes depicted corpulent females with full, rounded hips, but they were usually pregnant. In cave paintings dated to 30,000 years ago in Europe and in Africa, all the human figures are slender. There are no obese individuals, even among the royalty, on the wall paintings of Egyptian tombs.

Many Americans diet to improve their appearance, not their health. There is a stigma associated with obesity that results in poor community acceptance and lower employability. Television and magazine ads tend to portray obese persons deprecatingly. Insurance programs rank obesity as a risk factor, consistent with the finding that it may be responsible for up to 9.4 percent of health care costs in the United States.

The social pressure that induces overweight individuals to take off excess pounds may be diminishing. For one thing, they are clearly the majority in the U.S. population; more than half of us are overweight. Organizations lobby against discrimination toward the obese, especially that which is job-related. Perhaps the most ominous development is the finding by pediatric researchers at the University of Chicago. They noted that in low-income households, mothers did not consider their preschool children to be overweight unless they "could not move around or they were teased by other children." If parents think that being overweight is normal it will be difficult to slow down the rising rates of obesity and its complications anytime soon.

Of the thousand-plus diet programs available, almost all are based on a reduction in daily calorie intake. Some authors argue for a shift in the proportion of carbohydrate, protein and fat, even though scientific studies show that weight loss is independent of diet composition. Fat-burning pills, potions and foods are increasing in popularity, even as the rate of obesity climbs by almost 1 percent per year. Behavior barriers contribute to the difficulty of losing weight. Three of the most important are the Sacrifice Mentality, Calorie-Counter's Confusion and the Multiple Choice Dilemma.

The sacrifice mentality

One cannot cut calories significantly without sacrificing high-calorie favorite foods. Starting a 1,200-calorie diet means avoiding fast-food establishments, where a single meal can easily total 800 or 1,000 calories. Some desserts contain even more than that. Portion size can make some low-calorie diets downright disheartening. No wonder recidivism is the rule.

Calorie restriction of this degree inevitably leads to hunger, resentment and cravings. People on a diet lose control when they are famished. A person with a "hunger headache" can justify eating anything, even a handful of Oreo cookies, only 5 of which will provide 350 calories, produce a spike in blood sugar and yield a subsequent letdown. And the hunger will return in an hour or two. Lack of energy and irritability are two common complaints from calorie-restricted diets and, as might be expected, lead to binges and surrender. From a biological point of view, this is exactly what Nature intended. Survival depends on doing whatever it takes to provide energy.

We must expect cravings on a severely calorie-restricted diet because they are part of the normal survival mechanism. When we satisfy a craving by eating, it causes the release of serotonin, a hormone that produces a calming effect and helps to induce normal sleep. Nature did not intend for Sam and Sal to be able to resist cravings. Dieters don't realize that their response is quite normal, but collapse of their resolve leads to feelings of failure and eventual abandonment of the weight-loss program.

Lack of energy is common in dieters because in order to burn off fat they must first deplete the body's reserve of glycogen. This is the supply of short-term energy that we store in the liver and muscles.

Without these reserves it is impossible to maintain high-intensity physical activity. Dieters become dizzy for the same reason; there may be insufficient blood sugar (glucose) to nourish the brain. When both these conditions occur repeatedly it's easy to decide that losing a few pounds isn't worth the sacrifice.

Those who live with dieters often notice another side effect: halitosis, or bad breath. This is especially true in persons on a high-protein, high-fat, low carbohydrate diet. When the body breaks down fat for energy, it produces chemicals known as ketone bodies that it uses in place of glucose. These same ketone bodies form in diabetics whose disease is not in control. They produce an unpleasant odor and a characteristic "fruity" breath that experienced physicians recognize easily.

Some side effects of dieting are more subtle: dehydration and constipation. Dehydration occurs when individuals fail to maintain adequate fluid intake. They may not be aware that fasting is much more tolerable if one's fluid intake remains high. In fact, what is perceived as hunger is often thirst. As persons age they have a diminution in the sensation of thirst, and their risk of dehydration increases. Dieting certainly increases the risk.

Low fiber intake is characteristic of many calorie-restricting diets, and constipation is the inevitable result. Sam and Sal took in more than 100 grams of fiber a day. The average American takes in less than 20; a dieter may take in a fraction of that. It didn't take long for the laxative makers to spot an opportunity. You have probably seen the ads for Procter and Gamble and others who offer a "zero-carb solution to a low-carb problem."

Skipping meals, especially breakfast, is probably the most common casual method by which people try to lose weight. It is not only nonproductive, it is counterproductive. A study done at Vanderbilt University showed that those who skipped breakfast lost less weight in a monitored program than those who did not.

Breakfast-skippers were more likely to have a high-sugar, high-fat, mid-morning snack. The overnight fast leaves us with shallow reserves of glycogen. If we don't replenish our glycogen stores with an adequate breakfast we'll be hungrier during the day and will be more likely to succumb to the temptation of junk food.

Persons who skip breakfast function less well than breakfast-eaters. This is true at all ages. School performance is better among children who eat breakfast compared with those who do not.

If we skip one or two meals we may justify having a large meal late in the day. But the calories we take in during an evening meal are more likely to be stored as fat. This is because we don't have enough physical activity after that meal to use up those calories.

Calorie-counter's confusion

It is not possible to count calories accurately, and scores of studies prove that. As one researcher put it, "Having highly motivated volunteers is no guarantee of valid dietary reporting." When researchers asked a group of subjects to count the number of calories they took in over several days, they found large errors in the direction of undercounting. These were individuals who knew that they were being evaluated, yet they came up with implausible records. The typical underreporting error is about 20 percent. In some studies it is as high as 50 percent.

In order to count calories accurately we must use a food scale and a measuring cup — no estimates allowed. But we pour cereal from a box, not from a measuring cup, perhaps a little more today than we did yesterday. Today's banana might be half the size of tomorrow's. At the all-you-can-eat restaurant you might take one spoonful of potato salad; I might take two or three. Two tablespoons of salad dressing can easily add another 150 calories.

I do not intend to imply that we should not be concerned about the calorie content of various foods. It helps to know the approximate number of calories in common foods so that you can avoid those that are calorie-dense. It's easy to do this when you have made a habit of reading the Nutrition Information on packaged food. You'll notice that serving sizes can be surprisingly small. For instance, there are roughly 250 calories in a single slice of cheese pizza. A serving of Oreo crème-filled chocolate cookies (140 calories) consists of only two cookies.

Finally, even if we could accurately estimate calorie intake, how do we allow for differences in calories expended? The variations in our day-to-day activity negate any attempt to measure calories accurately. The person who walks at a moderate pace for thirty minutes will use about 100 calories more than the individual who watches TV for that same length of time. That represents a pound of fat that could have been lost by the TV-watcher, every 5 weeks!

> Most people count calories after the food is prepared. That's backward! Start with food that is low in calories and eat as much as you want.

The multiple choice dilemma

What proportion of our daily intake should consist of carbohydrate, protein and fat? The current Recommended Dietary Allowance (RDA) for carbohydrate is 55 percent, protein 15 percent and fat, no more than 30 percent. Sam and Sal ate more protein and less fat, a nutrient profile similar to that of most modern hunter-gatherers. Westerners take in more fat, more carbohydrate and less protein than the RDA. Promoters of diet programs advocate choices that are contradictory and contribute to the confusion of those who are trying to make healthy lifestyle changes. For example, the Protein Power diet has a fat content of 54 percent, Atkins 53 percent, the

Zone diet 33 percent and Sugar Busters 21 percent. Alleged experts have designed them but they may pose significant health risks. It may be a mixed blessing that few people stay on these diets for long. The reported attrition rate for the low-carbohydrate, high-protein diet is 43 percent, for the Zone diet 60 percent, and for a conventional low-calorie diet, 36 perent. There have been no published studies on the long-term consequences of low-carbohydrate, high-fat, high-protein diets, but in the short term they appear to increase the risk of kidney stones and osteoporosis.

Experts who warn against improper combining of macronutrients (carbohydrate, protein and fat) overlook the simple fact that early humans ate what was available. Natural foods contain a mixture of these macronutrients. The claim that adverse combinations confuse our enzyme systems is simply nonsense. Enzymes work when their substrate (their raw material) is present.

Sam and Sal thrived because of their lifestyle, not in spite of it. The proportion of carbohydrate, protein and fat in their diet was not critical because all their food sources had ample amounts of these. Remember

Are Eskimos fat? Only in cartoons. Underneath that bulky clothing is a slender body. If they eat no fruits or vegetables, where does their vitamin C come from? The answer is organ meats such as brain and kidney, and seafood.

that they had no large, juicy apples or softball-sized potatoes full of starch. Their fish and fowl were lean, and what fat these creatures did have was not saturated, like that in prime beef. They instinctively followed a biological maxim: eat to satiety and work (exercise) as life demands. That advice wouldn't work for us today. We must also adjust our diet to avoid what is inappropriate for our genetic endowment, supplement what is not naturally present in our food supply and exercise sufficiently to match our intake. Food selection does not have to be an agonizing mathematical exercise. I will discuss this in Chapter Six, Supermarket Suicide and Restaurant Roulette.

There was an enormous range of diets among pre-agricultural humans, as there is today among modern hunter-gatherers. Some of the latter are mostly vegetarian and have meat only occasionally. The Masai of sub-Saharan Africa live almost entirely on milk, blood and animal protein. In the Arctic, the only vegetables come from the stomachs of the animals they kill and some summertime mosses and lichens. No matter how varied their diets may be, these groups all share some common features: those who survive to old age are slender and strong, and they have almost no hypertension, diabetes, strokes or coronary artery disease. They do not develop these so-called age-related diseases until they take up a Western lifestyle.

Low-carbohydrate diets: more than a fad, less than a solution

The makers of bread, beer, donuts and desserts have been frantically redesigning their offerings ever since reputable medical journals published seemingly favorable results of low-carbohydrate diets. An enthusiastic popular press overlooked some key points. The initial studies were short-term, none lasting more than 12 months. Weight loss was modest. Few overweight subjects lost more than 10 percent of their starting weight and in one low-carbohydrate group the average weight loss was 3.4 percent at the end of the year. The dropout rate was sometimes greater than 40 percent. Approximately half the weight loss consisted of fat. The remainder represented muscle and other healthy tissue, known as lean body mass. Other studies show that so-called low-carb dieters take in more than twice the recommended level of carbohydrate, and very few remain in ketosis, said to be the fat-burning stage, for more than a few weeks.

Physicians who oppose low-carbohydrate programs are concerned about the long-term consequences of a diet that is high in saturated fat. In a welcome surprise, "bad" cholesterol hasn't risen as much, nor has "good" cholesterol declined as much as some had feared. That doesn't resolve all their doubts. For several decades, physicians have had moderate success with high-fat, low-carbohydrate diets in children with convulsions that cannot be controlled with the usual drugs. Contrary to the reassuring studies in adults, children do show changes in cholesterol and related substances that promote coronary artery disease. Some children on such a ketogenic diet develop heart abnormalities that disappear when they return to a normal diet.

It's likely that this fear-of-fat issue will disappear when polyunsaturated (omega-3s from fish) and monounsaturated (from olive oil) fats replace saturated (animal) fats and trans fats in low-carbohydrate programs. But it won't be anytime soon.

It's possible that neither the low carbohydrates nor the increased fats are what we should worry about, but a combination of these factors with a high protein intake. About 5 to 8 percent of children on a low-carbohydrate, high-fat diet develop kidney stones, a condition that pediatricians otherwise almost never see except in children with unusual genetic defects.

A reduced intake of fruits and vegetables is another concern, especially since the past two decades of research have shown so convincingly the protective effects of these foods against cancer and heart disease.

Low-carbohydrate diets work because they are also low calorie. The initial weight loss occurs as severe carbohydrate restriction depletes the muscles and liver of glycogen within a day or two. For every ounce of glycogen that we burn off as energy we eliminate three to five ounces of water. The average 150-pound person stores about 1 to 1½ pounds of glycogen and thus can expect to lose 4 to 8 pounds of weight in the first few days. None of this is fat, but it is encouraging to anyone who has a weight problem.

I suggest that persons who insist on going low-carb keep their protein intake at the pre-diet level. Protein helps to suppress appetite, which makes the low-carb diet easier to endure than most other low-calorie programs. Maintaining a normal intake of protein is good because it minimizes the loss of lean body mass, although not all studies confirm its protective effect.

Anyone that has lived with a person on a strict, low-calorie diet may have been aware of some personality changes. In a study of female cyclists, only one week of a low-carbohydrate diet resulted in increased levels of anger, tension and depression.

In spite of all this, there is some good that may come of the low-carb mania.

If Americans begin to realize that obesity is a threat to our economy as well as our health, and they can do something about it, we may finally be approaching the peak of the obesity epidemic. The food industry and government bodies are no longer ignoring this enormous problem. Junk food is slowly beginning to disappear from school cafeterias and some states have banned soft drinks from vending machines in schools.

Two Hershey's chocolate Kisses contain about 50 calories. So does a small apple or a medium-sized handful of broccoli. The chocolate is calorie-dense and has no vitamins, minerals or fiber, but it has lots of fat. The apple and broccoli have plenty of fiber, vitamins, minerals, a little protein, and no fat. So why couldn't God make broccoli taste like chocolate?

Another benefit of all this interest in low-carbohydrate meals is an awareness of carbohydrates in general. I'll discuss this in more detail in Chapter Five.

Promoters of low-carbohydrate diets have somehow overlooked a very significant fact: the populations of Okinawa and certain areas of the Mediterranean basin are the leanest, fittest and longest-lived on the planet, yet they thrive on diets that consist of more than 50 percent carbohydrate and very little fat. I'll discuss these further in Chapter Nine.

Is nature unfair to women?

If unwanted weight were the only thing that mattered, the answer would be an unequivocal "Yes!" Every husband and wife who have dieted and exercised together know that a man loses weight faster and with less effort than a woman. It makes men feel smug and frustrates women. But from a purely biological view, this gives women a significant advantage. There are two reasons, both rooted in natural selection. Women's bodies have evolved with certain physiologic characteristics that protect the infants they bear; the design of men's bodies enhances their role as hunters.

I've never heard a woman's portliness described as a beer belly, never heard a man called thunder thighs. These are gender-specific appellations, and they have a biological basis. Men accumulate fat primarily in the abdominal area; women deposit fat around the hips. They are referred to respectively as apples and pears, and only when obesity becomes pronounced do these distinctions disappear.

Men accumulate fat around the waist very easily, and can take it off almost as easily with moderate exercise and a correspondingly moderate reduction of food intake. This is hunter's fat, a store of energy that Sam did not have to carry on his back, was not subject to theft by other hunters or by vermin, and that did not interfere with running or throwing. During the two million years of our ancestral journey, from gathering fruit to chasing down game, males acquired this bodily trait that still persists but is no longer needed. The ancient advantages of abdominal fat, known to physicians as visceral fat, are countered by a serious disadvantage in the present day. Men easily accumulate visceral fat, which is deposited around internal abdominal organs, especially the loops of the intestine. Even when visceral fat is not obvious, it is associated with an increased risk of heart disease, high blood pressure, stroke and diabetes. Women also accumulate abdominal fat as their BMI increases. It carries with it the same high risk of cardiovascular disease that it does in men. The single most common cause of death in women is not breast cancer, it is atherosclerosis, which includes heart disease, stroke and hypertension.

Women normally have a higher percentage of body fat than men. Thigh fat accumulates quickly and is slow to disappear, as every woman knows. These facts are directly related to woman's role as child-bearer. Men can lower their percentage of body fat to 10 percent or less yet suffer few consequences as long as they remain fit and properly nourished. (Tiger Woods claims to have a body fat of 5 percent.) Women whose body fat percentage falls that low stop having menstrual periods and are unable to conceive. Those who do become pregnant produce breastmilk of poor quality. During the Dutch famine near the end of World War II, fertility rates declined. They returned to normal when the famine ended. This reduction in fertility is a survival mechanism. Fewer mouths to feed means less stress on the family unit. Women are understandably unhappy with the fat on their thighs, but if it were within and around the abdomen it would interfere with an enlarging uterus. On the other hand, a man with fat thighs couldn't run as fast, and if that fat were mobilized as slowly as it is in a woman, it wouldn't serve as well as a readily available store of energy.

Women's greater percentage of fat and slower mobilization of it probably have a role in survival under the most threatening conditions — prolonged starvation. Two million or so years ago the antecedents of Sam and Sal, known as Homo erectus, had neither the tools nor the creativity and adaptability of later hominids. They existed in small groups as most anthropoid species do today. Such a band could tolerate the loss of all but one or two of its males and still reproduce and survive. If only one or two females and several males survived, the perils of ordinary existence, the risks of pregnancy and childbirth, and high infant mortality would severely limit the chances that the band would continue to exist. Therefore,

> *Every schoolchild knows that Neanderthals also lived in the Stone Age. Most have not heard of Homo ergaster, Homo rudolfensis or Homo antecessor. These were members of our family tree that did not survive the primitive perils of prehistory. Perhaps their fat-storage capabilities were not as well developed as Homo sapiens'.*

woman's tendency to gain fat easily and to lose it only with difficulty is a biological victory. In the past half century it has become a biological liability.

Overcoming affluent malnutrition

It is not exaggeration to say that we are witnessing an epidemic of obesity and one of its main complications, diabetes. Since the 1970s the increase in both these conditions has been steady and costly. The rate of obesity in the United States is about 30 percent, but it is not only an American problem. It has doubled in the United Kingdom since 1980 and the rate of obesity is higher in several European countries than it is in the United States. It has tripled in China since 1990. Some Polynesian groups have rates of obesity exceeding 80 percent.

Obesity and its complications are rare in pre-contact aboriginal peoples just as they were almost certainly nonexistent before the advent of agriculture. It's clear from the work of Dr. Dean Ornish, Dr. John MacDougall and others that we can forestall and sometimes reverse coronary artery disease with a regimen of diet, exercise and stress reduction. Dr. Kenneth Cooper's studies reveal that individuals who exercise sufficiently can lower their risk of coronary events even though their body fat percentage remains higher than normal. Lowering the rates of obesity, diabetes and cardiovascular disease is a theoretically attainable goal, but the factors that militate against it are immense. Fat tastes good, sugar is everywhere and exercise is a bother. Knowledge of what our bodies are designed for is a beginning. It behooves us to design a simple but compelling strategy to help mankind reverse the problems we have brought upon ourselves by our affluence and abundance. The first step, literally, begins in Chapter Four.

Four

You have a genetic tendency toward exercise

PHYSICAL ACTIVITY IS an inborn genetic requirement for health and survival.

Under an intense African sun, a cheetah pursues a frantic antelope across the savannah. This drama is a matter of survival for both creatures. To our ancestors, escape and pursuit, as well as scores of less stressful daily activities, were also crucial for survival. They migrated, gathered, lifted, chopped, carried and climbed from the earliest age possible. These activities gave them a stronger cardiovascular and musculoskeletal system so that they could migrate farther, gather more, lift heavier loads and climb faster.

Most modern humans do not exercise as if their lives depended on it — but they do. No less than our ancient ancestors, those of us who migrate by car or plane, gather with the help of deliverymen, and lift nothing much heavier than a TV remote control device need to maintain our strength and endurance. The reasons are simple. If we do not use muscles they become smaller and weaker. If muscle force does not tax bones they become thinner, lighter, and more fragile. If we don't push our heart and lungs toward their limits they will have little reserve, incapable of meeting the demands of stress, infection or injury.

Thousands of generations ago the man or woman who did not exercise because of age or infirmity might become another creature's meal. Now, those of us who avoid accidental death are just as surely killed by diseases that were almost nonexistent, even in the elderly, back in prehistory. Instead of a death that came in seconds, however grisly those last seconds must have been, our dying takes years. The misery of leg pains from diabetic nerve degeneration or severely narrowed blood vessels, the tragedy of stroke, the energy drain of heart failure and the agony of the last stages of lung and other cancers are hardly more merciful than the swift ways in which our prehistoric ancestors died.

Long before the Agricultural Revolution made larger communities possible, Sam and Sal lived in small bands of perhaps 15 or 20 individuals. Most were always nomadic. Even where food was abundant it required ranging for at least a few miles almost every day, just as modern hunter-gatherers do. For most of Homo sapiens' existence as a species, and certainly during the long period when there were no real tools or controlled fire, storing food was not an option. Preservation techniques such as salting, drying and smoking are relatively recent, sometimes accidental, discoveries. Sam and Sal gathered food as primates do now, only enough for daily needs. Collecting fruits, vegetables, roots and nuts sometimes required a few miles of walking. They ran after game for even longer distances, sometimes for hours at a time. Most of us moderns find it hard to believe that a human has greater endurance than a deer. Our ancestors, as well as some hunter-gatherers of this century, could chase game animals until they slowed down from exhaustion, when they could approach and kill them easily.

Sam and Sal had only crude tools and no vehicles. Their strenuous way of life is evident in fossil skeletons, which have large, thick bones, especially at muscle attachments.

Aging does not cause osteoporosis; disuse of muscle leads to loss of muscle mass, then bone mass. Muscles become smaller if they are used infrequently and have little demand placed on them. Bone does the same, developing the thinned, sparsely calcified condition known as osteoporosis. In population groups where strenuous physical activity occurs well into middle age and beyond, neither muscle nor bone undergoes the diminution in size and strength that is obvious in the elderly of industrialized nations.

The Agricultural Revolution was probably the single most significant change in the socioeconomic landscape of the human species. When man learned to direct food production by sowing seed and reaping a harvest, and by taming and selectively breeding animals to yield meat and dairy products, he altered evolutionary patterns on a huge scale. There is no question that the benefits of agriculture, among which we include animal husbandry, are monumental, but strictly in terms of biology, so are the penalties.

The transition from wandering bands to fixed villages was only a temporary stage. As farming methods improved, small settlements became towns, then cities. The most highly developed agricultural economies were able to support armies to protect and conquer, and required a ruling elite.

Although the largest segment of the population continued to exercise strenuously as food producers, specialization of labor progressed and physical activity decreased for certain individuals. Masons and carpenters continued to use heavy hand tools, but priests and scribes did not. Porters and smiths needed all the muscle power of their distant hunter-gatherer ancestors, but merchants and weavers did not. Almost everyone lacked wheeled transportation or animals that they could ride, but as the millennia passed, all but the poorest peasants eventually walked less and less.

We only need to go back to the beginning of the twentieth century and compare it with the twenty-first to see a profound decline in our physical activity. Modern Americans are 75 percent less physically active than those who lived barely 100 years previously. Not too many years ago many families pumped water from wells by hand. The clerks who pulled food containers from the shelf one item at a time for waiting customers disappeared barely three generations ago, when supermarkets transformed the grocery business. Modern carpenters use power tools for almost every task.

How much progress can we afford?

Just as the Agricultural Revolution extracted a price, so did the Industrial Revolution. Dr. Frank Booth of the University of Missouri reduced it to its most basic essence: "Human cells are maladapted to an inactive lifestyle." The vital statistics of every economically advanced nation confirm it. All the chronic diseases of modern life are avoidable, and it is physical inactivity, along with our biologically bizarre food habits and use of tobacco (the leading cause of preventable death), that is to blame for many of them. The reasons will become clear in the pages that follow.

Muscle loss starts early

Have you ever noticed that old people shuffle? Why do you think they do that? It's because they just don't have enough energy to pick up their feet! Persons who shuffle trip easily. Of people over the age of 65, a full 25 percent cannot bathe themselves or dress themselves or feed themselves or even get out of bed without help. For those over the age of 85, more than 50 percent can't do those things. Those who can't get out of bed without someone to help are likely to fall when they try to do it alone, and a fall can be life-threatening in the elderly. We could avoid all those problems if we maintained our muscle mass with work or exercise instead of letting it diminish from disuse. After the age of 25, the average person loses muscle at the rate of about one-half of one percent a year, and that almost doubles after the age of 45.

Most people believe that our muscles inevitably become smaller as we age, although fitness mavens such as Bill Pearl and Jack Lalanne proved that this is not so. What actually happens is starkly evident to anyone who has had the misfortune of having fractured an arm or leg. When an extremity is immobilized for 4 or 6 weeks, the muscles shrink dramatically. It sometimes takes a great deal of commitment and expert physical therapy to restore those muscles to their original size and strength.

What happens in 6 weeks under a cast happens in 3 or 4 decades to the average person. But muscle mass does not have to decrease with age. For example, Bill Pearl became Mr. Southern California in 1953, at the age of 23. He won the Mr. Universe title 18 years later, at age 41, when most athletes are considered to be over the hill. In his late sixties, he still looked like he did in his forties.

Just as Sam and Sal's feeding habits were optimal for their physiologic makeup, so were their activity patterns. The heart and lungs, if they are conditioned by vigorous, prolonged activity, have a reserve that can be called upon in times of physical danger or infectious diseases. A well-developed muscular system is more than a source of power. The musculature of the arms and legs also acts as a pump to help the heart return blood to the lungs for a new supply of oxygen. Sluggish blood return is not usually serious, although the formation of blood clots in the legs is an often fatal complication of prolonged bed confinement. We can avoid unsightly varicose veins and painful hemorrhoids by keeping our leg muscles well toned.

Decreased physical activity is one of the most serious deviations we have made from our distant ancestral lifestyle. Barely 10 percent of Americans regularly engage in intense physical activity. The advances brought by the Industrial Revolution and the ubiquity of labor-saving devices have led to an inactivity epidemic that we can only halt by restoring normal activity levels. Exercise is the modern equivalent of day-to-day work of recent centuries. Survival demanded much physical exertion thousands of generations ago. Exercise, our substitute for work, is only an imitation of Stone Age activity, and has two components that are not equivalent to each other. These are anaerobic and aerobic exercise. I prefer to use the term resistance exercise in place of anaerobic in order to avoid confusion.

Anyone who starts an exercise routine for the first time, even a modest one, should have a thorough physical examination by a physician or other medical practitioner. For those who are under a physician's care, or who have had a thorough examination in the recent past, a special exam just for this purpose is not necessary. It is simply prudent to have periodic medical examinations in order to uncover disorders of recent onset such as high blood pressure and potentially serious heart abnormalities. When the famed runner, Jim Fixx, died suddenly at the age of 52, shortly after starting his daily run, an autopsy revealed that he had a cardiac abnormality which might have been identified with an ordinary physical examination. This is not unusual. Hypertension as well as abnormalities of the heart valves and coronary arteries can be present without symptoms.

Get a physician's clearance to exercise if you:

- are over the age of 40
- have diabetes
- have a history of heart disease
- have a history of fainting
- have had chest pain during exercise
- plan to engage in competitive exercise
- have not had a physical examination in the past two years or if anyone in your family has died suddenly before the age of 40

A second reason is more motivational than medical. Aerobic and resistance exercises bring significant physiological and chemical changes within a relatively short time. As you watch your pulse rate, blood pressure and blood cholesterol decline you'll feel a great sense of accomplishment, but in order to do that you'll need to know from where you started — your baseline measurements.

In the several million years of evolution between early anthropoids and modern man, Nature devised an exquisite interrelationship between our environment and our body chemistry. In the healing of a wound injury, for example, there are dozens of interrelated chemical actions, and probably hundreds we haven't discovered yet. Exercise enhances production of specific substances that reduce the inflammation that occurs when a portion of heart muscle is injured, and other chemicals that protect the heart when it receives less oxygen. Exercise also alters the nervous system so that when a heart attack occurs, there is less likelihood that a fatal abnormality of the heart rhythm will occur.

No exercise or no food. The results are eventually the same.

If you stop eating entirely:
- *The body gets lighter as fat, then protein, are used for energy.*
- *Vital organs, including the brain, don't work as well.*
- *When muscle mass decreases, daily chores become impossible.*
- *Immune function deteriorates as critical protein is used up.*
- *Death occurs quickly.*

If you stop exercising entirely:
- *The body gets lighter as unused muscles and bones waste away.*
- *Vital organs, especially the brain, don't work as well.*
- *When muscle mass decreases, daily chores become impossible.*
- *Immune function deteriorates as exercise-dependent hormonal factors diminish and the body loses valuable protein stores.*
- *Death occurs slowly.*

Aerobic exercise — taking the first steps

Aerobic exercise is that which requires oxygen, and occurs over at least several minutes. For example, you can hold your breath to run half a block (anaerobic), but not half a mile (aerobic). There are several kinds of aerobic exercises, including walking, running, cross-country skiing, cycling, rowing, swimming, etc., all of which a trained athlete can maintain for hours. For the average person, walking is the best choice. Other kinds of aerobic exercise are relatively inconvenient. Running is a good example. It requires special shoes and is seldom done in street clothes. Unless a track or treadmill is nearby you'll have to accept neighborhood traffic and hard pavement. Stress fractures occur with some frequency in runners, and even in those who are well-conditioned, knee and hip disorders are much more common than in walkers. The special equipment and conditions of the other exercises mentioned above are self-evident.

For the beginning walker it's important to start with a slow pace and a short distance. Five minutes may be just the right duration for some beginners; an hour is probably too long for any beginner. Extending the duration of the walk by about 5 minutes each day is enough to get to the desired objective, about 30 to 45 minutes, in less than two weeks. Plan on doing it 3 to 5 times a week.

The best pace is roughly 3 to 4 miles per hour, so that you can comfortably engage in conversation during the entire walk. Some fitness experts recommend interval training or wind sprints, in which you speed up the activity for one or two minutes before resuming the regular pace. This results in slight gains in conditioning as well as in fat burning. It isn't necessary to walk very fast or to run in order to burn fat calories. The rate of fat utilization in running is only about 15 percent greater than that for moderate walking for a given period of time, and the hazards of running increase disproportionately.

Compared with walking, vigorous activity does not offer a significant advantage in lowering the risk of heart disease.

There is no best place to walk. It's a matter of what is convenient enough so that you will be willing to do it 3 or 4 times a week. An exercise treadmill, either in the home or at a fitness center, is the most convenient if weather is a factor. As price and sophistication increase, these machines provide a variety of speeds and inclines, a choice of programs, and a display of the distance covered, speed, heart rate, calories burned, etc. If you take special delight in having company and enjoying scenery while exercising, a lonely treadmill is a poor substitute for walking with a friend in a park or neighborhood.

If a treadmill has a display panel which indicates time, speed, slope, distance, expended calories and heart rate, it's easy to set personal achievement goals which can be so motivating that you'll look forward to each session. Within weeks of starting you'll record speeds and incline settings that you would not have thought possible in the first few days.

Although casual clothing is quite adequate, ordinary shoes might not be. Quality walking shoes are a wise investment, not just for comfort, but also for foot health. Anyone with preexisting foot problems should seek out those shoe or sporting goods stores which provide professional advice as well as quality footwear. Most podiatrists and sports medicine specialists can recommend the best ones.

Warming up and cooling down are part of any exercise routine, whether of the aerobic or resistance type. Muscles are laced with tiny blood vessels called capillaries that are not all open at the same time in a resting muscle. The warm-up, consisting of 3 to 5 minutes of brisk walking or light calisthenics, gradually opens up more of this network and increases blood flow so that when sudden demands are placed on the muscle, it will not be starved for oxygen and nutrients. A warm-up also helps to relax the tendons that attach muscle to bone, and the ligaments that connect bones to each other.

There may be some evolutionary reason for a warm-up. Sam and Sal were active most of the time; they were always "warmed up." Their muscles, ligaments and tendons were instantly available for the demands that a sudden spurt of activity put on them. Like animals in the wild (which they were) all their systems had to be ready to escape in an instant or pounce upon their prey. In a body that is warm, oxygen more readily passes from blood to muscle. Muscles that are warm work better than those that are not, and are more resistant to injury.

A cool-down period is just as important as the warm-up. After you have worked out, walk slowly until your heart rate is about 10 to 15 beats above its normal resting rate. Don't sit down or lie down immediately. Without a cooling-down period the heart rate decreases rapidly and blood tends to pool in the legs. This can affect the blood supply to the heart and could obviously be serious in someone with underlying heart disease.

Just as you should not stop exercising abruptly, you should wait about 20–30 minutes before taking a hot shower, bath or sauna. Each of these causes increased blood flow through the skin in a natural effort to lower body temperature. This diversion of blood from the brain and heart could possibly cause a sudden drop in blood pressure, fainting, or even a heart attack.

Developing an exercise routine is a challenge for many people, but there are some things you can do to make it easier to establish a lifelong habit pattern. A good aerobic schedule consists of 3 or 4 days per week for 30 to 45 minutes. If less time is available, or you can find only a few short segments of time, use what you have. All exercise is beneficial.

Seven easy steps to a walking routine

- Have a goal in mind. Decide on the number of days per week, number of hours, or miles walked.

Need a walking tool?
Try a pedometer.

A pedometer keeps track of the steps you take. It can motivate you to walk more by recording your activity so that you can see if you're close to your daily or weekly goal. Some units only measure steps. Others show miles and/or calories.

---

* Plan a schedule and make it part of your daily or weekly routine. The best time is usually in the morning, before breakfast. For those with a full-time job, lunchtime or immediately after work may be best. After dinner is not the best time for most people. Fatigue, a full stomach and family obligations can quickly dissolve good intentions.
* Find a partner. You can encourage each other and make the time go faster. Sometimes it's a help to be responsible to another person when the weather is marginal or you just are not in the mood for exercise.
* If you walk alone, use CDs or cassette tapes to relax or to learn, or to motivate yourself. Every library has hundreds of books on tape, and there's nothing quite like a resonant voice accompanying you during an otherwise boring session on a treadmill or step machine.
* If you walk through your neighborhood, vary your route. Boredom kills resolve.
* Keep safety in mind. When you walk alone, stay in areas where there will be someone who can assist you if you turn an ankle or have a more serious problem. Cell phones are so light, small and inexpensive that it's prudent to carry one no matter where you walk.
* Periodically set different goals for distance, time, speed, incline or pulse rate. Give yourself geographic goals. How

many days would it take you to walk from Boston to New York (216 miles) if you walked 2 ½ miles a day around your neighborhood? San Francisco to Los Angeles (403 miles)? Paris to Vienna (560 miles)? Reward yourself when you reach a goal — but not with chocolate!

Avoid pitfalls

There is no sport or exercise without pitfalls. Walking probably has the fewest, but be mindful of these:

- Don't push yourself too far, especially in the early days. Keep things in perspective. You are going to be exercising for many years. Taking a couple of weeks to get up to your desired pace and distance is very reasonable. If you overdo it you'll develop muscle soreness, one of the most common reasons why beginners give up exercising.
- Keep up your fluid intake. The older you are, the less reliable is your thirst mechanism. Unless you are walking for a short time in cool weather, carry water or an electrolyte-containing drink with you and sip frequently. Sports drinks are not necessary for casual activity that lasts for no more than 30 or 45 minutes, but those who walk longer should keep up with both fluids and electrolytes.
- Dress appropriately. Specifically, do not wear occlusive clothing that inhibits natural cooling. Plastic exercise suits are especially dangerous. Excessive sweating leads to loss of water and salt that can result in heat exhaustion, a serious matter.
- Be aware of traffic hazards, especially if you walk while wearing headphones. Obey traffic signals and be aware that a driver may not be prepared to adjust his or her usual scan to

accommodate a pedestrian who is running or walking fast. As an extra precaution, stay as far from traffic lanes as possible in order to avoid the occasional intoxicated or distracted driver who may drift out of a lane.

- Avoid walking at night, if possible. Irregular pavement surfaces and other ankle-turning hazards may not be obvious. If walking during daylight hours is not an option, avoid routes that will take you across busy streets. Wear light-colored clothing and apply reflective strips to your cap, jacket, pants and shoes. Reflective material is available at most sporting goods stores. Women should not walk alone after dark. If you must walk at night, do so where there will be other persons who can help you in case of a fall or other accident.
- Wear sunscreen and proper covering even on overcast days. Clouds won't protect you from being harmed by ultraviolet rays.
- If you are diabetic, be sure to ask your physician about ways to protect your feet, and how to recognize small injuries that heal poorly and become easily infected. Persons with diabetes should select footwear carefully, maintain good foot hygiene and get prompt medical attention for any skin injury that does not heal quickly.
- A treadmill is an unforgiving machine. Never put on headphones or adjust a radio or recording device when the belt is moving. Most treadmills have a safety cord that will stop the machine in case you do fall.
- Hand weights may seem to increase the benefits of walking, but I don't recommend them. Using weights may cause back or shoulder injury.

Resistance exercise

When we push or pull against gravity we are doing resistance exercise. It doesn't necessarily mean lifting a barbell or pulling a cable or using an exercise machine. Raking leaves or making a bed, swinging a child or driving a golf ball, all help to maintain

> We don't do less because we lose muscle. We lose muscle because we do less.

our muscle mass. For the vast majority of us, however, these activities taken together don't add up to enough expenditure of energy to match what Nature designed our bodies for.

Muscle burns calories, even when you're asleep. Increasing your muscle mass is like setting your car's engine to a fast idle. It's burning fuel even though it's not going anywhere. People with lots of muscle can eat more and not get fat, because although they might be at rest, that muscle mass is burning calories.

Muscle is also a place where the body stores energy in the form of glycogen. The more muscle mass you have, the more glycogen you can store and have ready when you need it. That's one of the reasons people who exercise have more energy and feel better.

Muscle stores more than energy; it also holds a supply of protein that is available in times of stress.

> Muscle is 37 times more metabolically active than fat.

Diseases of the elderly, especially those of the heart and kidneys, drain the body of protein. Persons with a smaller mass of muscle are less able to withstand the loss of protein that accompanies illness, especially when it compromises their intake of wholesome food.

We can restore some lost muscle at any age, although the amount of muscle mass we're able to regain is influenced largely by age and the progressive decline in production of human growth hormone and testosterone. Researchers in Boston conducted a study in which residents of a convalescent home were put on a strength-training program. They called it "Old's Gym." The average age was 90.2 years. Eighty percent had a history of falls. They had an average of 4 chronic illnesses. But in 8 weeks, they had tripled their strength and increased their muscle mass by 10 percent. In as little as 2 months it's possible to regain the loss in strength and muscle mass that has occurred over 20 years. The message is very clear: you can respond to exercise at any age.

In other studies in which people over the age of 70 began weight-training exercises, the ones who couldn't get out of a wheelchair were able to walk without assistance. Those who couldn't walk down the hall soon were able to explore most of the facility. One study showed that men in their 70s who had been doing resistance exercises were as strong or stronger than the average 28-year-old who did not.

Heart disease is seldom a barrier to resistance exercise, especially in persons recovering from a heart attack. When properly supervised exercise actually reduces cardiac risk factors.

Avoiding sarcopenia

Sarcopenia means reduction in flesh. It is the diminution in skeletal muscle that was once thought to be a normal consequence of aging, but which we now know is mostly due to inactivity. Recent research is making it clear that several diseases of aging are directly related to this loss of muscle.

Diabetes

Animals in the wild don't get type 2 diabetes. Neither do hunter-gatherers, even if they have the gene for it. The Pima Indians (Chapter One) definitely have the gene for diabetes, but it is almost nonexistent in the Mexican Pimas. The conclusion of some researchers is that type 2 diabetes mellitus, known as adult-onset diabetes, is mostly an exercise-deficiency disease.

Obesity and the lack of exercise are indisputably linked to the development of adult-onset diabetes. When you exercise, you use up blood sugar, so the levels tend to stay lower and more constant. If blood sugar levels are consistently in the normal range, insulin levels also remain low. High insulin levels lead to insulin-resistance (Chapter Five), which ultimately leads to diabetes.

In a person of normal build, skeletal muscle accounts for about 40 percent of body weight. Since this muscle is where most insulin activity occurs, regular exercise that lowers blood sugar levels also lowers the risk of diabetes. Unfortunately for those with a fickle attitude toward fitness, it only takes a few days of physical inactivity to reverse the beneficial effects of exercise.

Persons with diabetes frequently develop skin ulcerations of the foot, which heal slowly and often become infected. Regular exercise improves the flow of blood through the skin and may prevent the formation of ulcers.

Osteoporosis

Exercise that increases muscle mass also increases bone density. Bone that is called upon to support a heavier load adapts by becoming thicker and heavier, especially at those points at which muscles are attached. When we reverse that mechanism by giving bone less to do it becomes thin and brittle. That's why resistance-type exercise helps to prevent the loss of bone that we call osteoporosis. Osteoporosis is not a disease of aging. It's a condition that results from lack of exercise. In women who exercised only two times a week, loss of bone was arrested after one year of study. In persons who did not exercise, bone loss continued during that same period.

Exercise is especially important in persons whose calcium intake is chronically low. Black South Africans and Melanesians have a calcium intake lower than that of most people in the United

> Wolff's Law: bone remodeling is directly dependent on the mechanical load placed on it. In other words, the more stress we place on our skeleton in the course of our daily lives, the stronger it will be.

States, but they have fewer fractures. Their unmechanized society demands much more physical activity. As a result, the cross-sectional shape of their bones is more oval instead of round, which lessens the risk of fracture.

Accidents

If you have strong muscles you won't lose your balance easily, and you will recover your balance better. Joint instability, for instance, is due to weakness of the muscles around a joint, not the joint itself. Stronger leg muscles help to stabilize the knee so that a twisting motion is less likely to result in a fall, or in a torn cartilage or ligament. Strengthening the upper body with resistance exercise leads to a lower risk of elbow and shoulder injury. Restoring the muscles of the abdomen and back will result in fewer back injuries and less back pain.

There is more to balance than strong, stabilizing muscles. Every muscle fiber contains sensitive nerve endings that constantly send signals to the brain, helping us to maintain balance by making continual adjustments in muscle tension. If we allow our muscles to waste away through inactivity, we lose some of the ability to keep our balance.

Weak muscles, loss of balance and thin bones are obviously a potentially life-threatening combination. Regular, demanding exercise can help persons of any age reduce the risk of falls.

Heart attack and stroke

Heart disease accounts for about 40 percent of all deaths in the United States. Lack of exercise is one of the most important contributors to this high rate through a variety of mechanisms.

When you have greater muscle mass your metabolic rate will be higher. That means more of what you eat is used up to provide energy instead of being converted to fat. Having less fat in your bloodstream makes it less likely that you will have a buildup of artery-clogging plaque in the arteries of your heart and brain. Increased blood pressure, heart attack and stroke rarely occur in pre-agricultural people, or in Americans who exercise consistently and vigorously. In persons whose blood pressure is at the upper limits of normal, strength training returns it to the normal range.

A heart attack takes years to develop. The earliest changes occur when a chronic lack of physical activity keeps the coronary arteries (the blood vessels that supply the heart muscle directly) from dilating periodically under the normal demands of work. Without this structural enlargement, these vessels cannot adapt to acute stress, and are less able to accommodate the build-up of artery-clogging materials that accumulate because of poor dietary habits.

Regular exercise also leads to the formation of *cardioprotectants*, chemical substances that limit muscle damage when blockage of an artery injures the heart. When physical activity is maintained on a chronic basis the body increases the level of other chemicals that promote good blood flow to the heart.

Eighty percent of strokes are due to obstruction of a blood vessel that nourishes a portion of the brain. Regular physical activity reduces the risk of this type of stroke by increasing levels of HDL (good) cholesterol, and by lowering the levels of several substances within the blood that increase clotting tendencies. Rupture of a blood vessel within the brain, often precipitated by high blood pressure, accounts for most of the other 20 percent of strokes. When an area within a blood vessel wall becomes weak, it bulges outward and forms an aneurysm. Regular exercise lowers blood pressure and thus reduces risk to some degree. There are multiple causes of blood vessel wall weakness, which include smoking, and exercise has little influence on this group.

Gallbladder disease

It seems like a long leap from muscle to gallbladder disease, but there are some plausible explanations for the observation that women who exercise for 2 or 3 hours a week lessen the risk of gallbladder surgery by about 20 percent. (Men have a much lower incidence of gallbladder disease than women do.)

Exercise lowers cholesterol levels, and this substance forms most gallstones. Even in the absence of obesity, some people become insulin-resistant, which also increases the risk. In persons who do not exercise, intestinal contents move more slowly, which makes gallbladder disease more likely.

Cancer

Some studies show that exercise reduces certain cancers, including melanoma, a serious form of skin cancer. The list includes cancer of the colon, prostate, breast and pancreas, but the explanations cover a wide array of factors. They range from the growth-promoting effects of insulin to immune function, as well as estrogen and testosterone activity.

The association of cancer and physical inactivity is not strong, but it is consistent, and illustrates the complex interaction of our body chemistry and exercise.

Insomnia

One of the most common complaints among the elderly is that they don't sleep well. This isn't due to aging, but to physical illness, medications and lack of exercise. Depression, heart disease, lung disease and upper airway problems are common in this age group, and they all can make getting restful sleep difficult. The need to get up at night to urinate also interferes with sleep. The elderly tend to stay indoors more than younger persons and lose some of the light-induced variation in body rhythm.

The usual recourse for insomnia, especially for older individuals, is a prescription for a sleep-inducing medication. This group of drugs is notorious for side effects, which include confusion, agitation and a heightened risk of falling, as well as daytime drowsiness and increased risk of auto accidents.

Exercise isn't an antidote for all these problems, but walking 4 times a week for 30 to 40 minutes does improve sleep patterns. People who exercise not only get to sleep twice as fast, but they sleep about one hour longer. Resistance exercise also helps. In an over-60 group in Boston, exercise routines directed at the larger muscle groups improved sleep quality, and relieved depression.

Some people avoid exercise late in the evening, worrying that it will interfere with a normal night's sleep. It will not. When researchers subjected a group of cyclists to intense exercise just before bedtime, they fell asleep just as quickly and slept as long as they did on those days when they didn't exercise.

Arthritis

Arthritis (osteoarthritis) of the knees is more likely to occur among people who are obese, and those with weak leg muscles. Strong muscles in the legs keep the knees more stable and provide a braking action so that the impact of the foot hitting the ground is not as forceful. Our knees don't simply wear out. Impact is what damages the cartilage, and the more muscle we have on both sides of a joint, the less severe the impact.

Replacement of arthritic knees is among the most common surgical procedures of the recent decade, and the upward trend can only continue as our population ages. Resistance training can do little for those whose disease is well established, but we can markedly reduce the likelihood of developing osteoarthritis and chronic joint injury with a relatively small increase of leg strength.

Exercise benefits those who already have osteoarthritis by maintaining flexibility and by improving muscle conditioning.

Glaucoma

Glaucoma is an eye disorder in which the pressure within the eyeball increases and damages delicate structures. It is the second most common cause of blindness in the United States, yet about half of those who have the disease are unaware of it. By the time a person develops changes in vision there has already been significant damage. There is no currently available treatment that can restore vision lost by glaucoma. Drugs that are used in the treatment of glaucoma have numerous side effects.

Eye specialists have known for some time that exercise, especially resistance-type exercise, lowers pressure within the eye. The decrease is even greater in patients with glaucoma than it is in normal persons. However, exercise at any level will not be a replacement for drugs or surgery in the treatment of glaucoma. No one knows if lifelong exercise can reduce the risk of glaucoma, but that's a benefit worth considering.

Brain function

You probably have noticed that you feel sharper and think more clearly when you do aerobic exercise. It's not just for the short term, and not just for the young. Moderate physical activity does more than just increase blood flow to the brain. In animal studies, exercise causes new brain cells to grow, and new connections between cells appear. We can't study people the same way, of course, but elderly persons who walk several days a week do better at tasks requiring attention than those who don't. That particular ability resides in a part of the brain where animal studies show new cell growth and richer interconnections. Regular exercise increases the level of acetylcholine, a critical neurotransmitter that allows impulses to spread from one brain cell to another, and is important in the memory process.

Muscle myths

There are a few myths regarding exercise, especially resistance exercise, which might deter some people from beginning a strength-training program.

Myth #1. Exercise needs to be strenuous. Unless you intend to engage in competitive sports or to become a bodybuilder, moderate exercise is all that is necessary to maintain fitness. In fact, one of the best ways to lose fat and to keep from accumulating more is to do some mild exercise on a daily basis while avoiding an excess calorie intake. Just a few routines using light weights are adequate. (See Appendix 2.)

Myth #2. I'll become musclebound. Ever since someone coined the term early in the twentieth century it has been difficult to find examples of this condition. It takes a long time, extraordinary effort, uncommon discipline and, often, supplementary hormones to develop the oversized muscles of competitive bodybuilders.

Myth #3. I'm too old. Remember our description of Old's Gym in Boston. There is no upper limit for exercising. You can be 100, and if you start to exercise you're going to get stronger.

How to get started with resistance exercise

The goal of a resistance exercise program is to increase or to maintain muscle mass. The term weight training is common even though machines and elastic bands can be used for resistance. Two or three days a week is all that is needed, preferably alternating with your aerobic schedule.

It's just as important to start slowly with resistance exercise as it is with aerobics.

Muscles that have been dormant will ache for days if we awaken them suddenly with strenuous activity. This is because a muscle will increase in size and strength only if it is temporarily damaged or injured by the stress put upon it. The recovery following such injury is what causes the muscle cell to become larger and stronger, ready for the next challenge.

We accomplish two objectives when we gradually increase the weight we use and the intensity of the exercise. First, the blood vessels that nourish an inactive muscle are accustomed to a small volume of blood. If we proceed gradually the body will enlarge these vessels and form new ones, but this will not occur instantaneously. An adequate blood supply will ensure that the muscles will receive sufficient amounts of oxygen and nutrients and will remove the by-products of muscle activity, lactic acid and carbon dioxide.

Second, a gradual approach minimizes pain and discomfort. If you have not been exercising I suggest that you go through the routine with no weights at all for a few sessions. You will not only avoid the aches which inevitably occur when subjecting muscles to new stress, but you will develop the proper form, which includes a full range of motion. You'll also find that even if you use no weights, your muscle tone will improve and you will feel more energetic.

When you lift any weight you need more than just muscle. Tendons attach muscles to bones; ligaments connect bones to each other. Both structures lose elasticity as we grow older and they can tear easily. It takes longer to get them in good condition than it takes for muscle, which has a much richer blood supply. Just because you feel strong enough to lift heavy weights doesn't mean that you should. Give your tendons and ligaments several weeks to get back in shape.

During this breaking-in period you can decide whether to work out at home or at a fitness center. You will need some equipment for a home exercise routine. Light dumbbells or elastic bands are perfectly adequate for the first few weeks or months, or even longer. A well-equipped home fitness room is a luxury, both in regard to expense and floor space, but if those issues are unimportant it can be well worth it. Every newspaper classified ad section offers exercise equipment for pennies on the dollar.

If a commercial fitness center is close by it may be the best place for both aerobic and resistance exercise. These facilities have several advantages, one of which is the availability of trainers who can guide you in the safe and effective use of the equipment.

Will electrostimulation of muscles replace hours in the gym?

Those who succumb to advertising for these devices fail to recognize the difference between stimulation of a muscle group and true exercise. Muscles grow and become stronger when they contract and relax under a stressful load. The relatively meager activity that occurs when a mild electrical impulse causes fibers to contract is no more likely to cause muscle growth than doing exercises with no resistance. The models in those television commercials got their large muscles the old-fashioned way: they worked for them.

For any given muscle group there are literally scores of exercises and techniques. One can use barbells, dumbbells, machines and elastic bands for most of them. There are different programs of instruction. Every individual will find some exercises and some machines that are comfortable and some that are not. There is only one universal dictum: everyone needs to do resistance exercises two or three times a week to avoid muscle wasting and its consequences. There is information on selecting exercise equipment in Appendix 1. In Appendix 2 you'll find a description of several basic exercises. For those readers who may be interested in more detailed exercise routines, there are useful references in Appendix 4.

About workouts

A single exercise movement, back and forth or up and down, is called a repetition (rep); two or more repetitions constitute a set; several sets make up a routine.

You don't need to exercise every muscle in your body individually. They work together in groups. Keep your routine varied in order to use all the muscles within a group.

Are you a greyhound or a St. Bernard?

Get to know your body type — and love it. I'm not referring to apple or pear shapes. Those body shapes are acquired, not inherited. Nature has endowed some of us with lanky body types that no amount of weight training will ever convert to a Mr. or Mrs. Universe contender. But then, those big-boned, muscular types that can lift three times their body weight at the Olympics would be at the back of the pack at the Boston marathon.

Don't confuse body type with body fat. We all know the skinny kid in high school who shows up at the 30-year reunion unable to see his toes without the aid of a mirror. If he had avoided excess calories and exercised every day he'd be in great shape — but still slender. Genetics determine how much muscle he could pack onto his light-boned frame, and chances are it wouldn't be very much. Some of us are just plain bulky, with heavy frames and chunky muscles, which with some training could qualify us for the next home town bodybuilding contest.

Here's a simple test. Place one hand around the opposite wrist and touch the tips of the thumb and middle finger together. If they can overlap you are light-boned. If they don't touch at all you have a heavy frame. Medium frame is obvious: the fingers touch lightly.

Light-framed persons are greyhound types. They have a predominance of slow-twitch muscle fibers that make them good long-distance runners. Big-boned St. Bernard types have a predominance of fast-twitch muscle fibers that allow them to make rapid lifting movements. The person of medium build has almost equal numbers of fast-twitch and slow-twitch muscle fibers, 55 and 45 percent, respectively. Competitive marathoners have as much as 82 percent slow-twitch fibers, and competitive swimmers 74 percent. No amount of training can change those ratios.

Interestingly, weightlifters don't have an excess of fast-twitch fibers. Their ratio, 55 to 45 percent, is the same as those with a medium build. Perhaps it's because the slow-twitch fibers cannot enlarge, whereas the fast-twitch fibers can. In other words, persons with the bone structure and muscle type of long-distance runners can never "bulk up," while those with medium or large frames can.

Whichever type you are, it's what you will be throughout your adult life, and no amount of exercise, special diets or supplements will ever change it. It's also no excuse for being overweight. Each of the three types can add 100 pounds or more of fat.

About pain

If you take a tour through your neighborhood fitness center you'll probably hear some grunts and groans when you pass the room lined with racks of barbells and dumbbells. Don't be discouraged or intimidated by the heavy-lifting, intensely focused men and women who look like they're not enjoying themselves at all. Concentrate on the not-so-muscled majority, whose lifting is less than Olympic and who socialize between sets. These are the Sams and Sals of your generation, folks who realize that they need to lift something heavier than the groceries a couple of times a week. They'll never be on the Mr. or Mrs. Olympia stage, but they'll enjoy another stage in life, the last, in which they will be self-sufficient and minimally burdened by chronic disease.

That's not to say that you won't encounter some soreness or discomfort from time to time, but it won't even come close to the pain of a fractured hip or the agony of a collapsed vertebra, the outcomes of osteoporosis. There's a difference between (a) the "burn" you'll experience after an intensive set of exercises, (b) the aching you might feel when you exercise muscles which you haven't used for some time (known as delayed onset muscle soreness) and (c) the pain of injury. A mild burning sensation may occur when you have done several repetitions of an exercise. This is not only normal, but it means that you have reached a level of intensity that is going to make that muscle grow. It lasts for no more than a few seconds. Another kind of pain is the slight — sometimes intense — muscle ache that occurs the day after working in the garden or trying to keep up with children in the playground. This is normal when we use muscles after a long period of inactivity. It produces the mild injury that results in subsequent growth. This delayed-onset soreness may take several days for recovery and you can avoid it, or at least reduce it, by following the guidelines given above.

> If a muscle has been dormant for two weeks or more you can expect some discomfort when you start exercising again. To avoid this after a period of inactivity, always start with lower weights than you used previously.

Pain is recognizably different from immediate burn and delayed soreness. It's a signal to stop exercising. Never try to "work it out." A torn ligament might take weeks or months to heal. If the pain is severe, if it lasts for more than a day, or if it recurs at the next workout session, obtain medical advice before resuming the exercise that induced it.

Don't take aspirin to relieve delayed onset soreness. A substance called prostaglandin E2 is important in muscle repair but aspirin inhibits its activity. Neither aspirin nor other common pain-relieving medications significantly reduce delayed-onset muscle soreness.

In a study from the United Kingdom, taking 400 milligrams of supplemental vitamin C for two weeks prior to starting an exercise routine appeared to reduce muscle soreness when compared with a placebo.

Get the most from your effort

Rest for about one minute between sets of exercises unless you have been instructed in a special routine. Always allow a minimum of 48 hours' rest between resistance exercise days. The slight injury that forces a muscle to grow takes time to heal and to build more muscle. Exercise that is too intense or too frequent is counterproductive and may lead to injury. Use the "off" day to walk or to rest completely.

Slower is better. Take at least 3 seconds for the positive phase of an exercise, in which you raise the weight. After a one-second pause, allow 3 or 4 seconds to lower the weight (the negative phase). By slowing down the movements you can use less weight to obtain the same benefit and reduce the risk of injury.

Don't cheat. Sudden, yanking movements and using leverage will help you to lift heavier weights, but will dramatically increase the risk of injury and it will reduce the benefit to the muscle group you are trying to strengthen. That rapid jerking motion you've seen during Olympic weight-lifting competition is not exercise.

A strict routine isn't necessary unless you have a specific training goal. Just be sure to involve all major muscle groups every week. (Appendix 2 illustrates a starting routine for the back, shoulders, chest, arms, legs and abdomen.) Training the upper and lower body on different days is as effective as working on all parts on the same day. It also makes each day's routine shorter and more convenient for the busy person.

Don't get into a rut. Vary your routine every couple of months. It will keep you motivated to continue.

Don't worry about who may be watching you exercise. Nobody cares about how much you can lift. Don't be embarrassed to use a barbell with no plates, the lightest dumbbells on the rack, or the lowest setting on a machine.

Always stretch at the end of your routine, when your muscles have become warm and relaxed. It's a good way to cool down and keeps you supple. Stretching techniques vary almost as much as exercise techniques. (See Appendix 4.)

Never try to see how much you can lift. It ranks near the top of the list of Stupid Ways to Injure Yourself.

If you lift heavy weights, always have a spotter, a companion who can help you out of a difficult, painful, or dangerous situation. Never bench press without having someone standing by.

Always monitor children closely when they do resistance exercises, especially adolescents. They need a routine designed specifically for their age as well as their stage of development, supervised by trained instructors or coaches. Peer pressure is intense, especially among young athletes, and trying to lift too much can result in lifelong injury.

> **Avoid these high-risk exercises:**
>
> - *Dead lift. It can cause serious back injury.*
> - *Sit-ups with feet anchored can also injure the back.*
> - *Bench press with barbell. A machine is safer.*
> - *Deep squats are a leading cause of knee injury.*
> - *Leg press with heavy weight can lead to knee damage.*
> - *Straight leg lifts while lying on your back.*
> - *Any shoulder exercise with heavy weights.*

Every fitness center, supermarket and health food store sells a tempting and expensive line of muscle-building supplements. Spectacular results are anecdotal and not backed by research; studies backed by research are not spectacular. Some of these supplements do work, but the increased benefit in controlled studies is generally in the range of about 5 percent. That's a small gain from a costly investment.

If you still need a good reason to start an exercise routine, or to continue it when you think you're not making progress, or time is at a premium, consider these benefits of regular exercise.

- Exercise lowers body fat without side effects
- Improves the way the body uses glucose (blood sugar) for energy
- Improves the shape of the body as fat disappears from the waist and hips and posture improves
- Center of gravity returns to normal, lowering risk of chronic back pain and back injury
- Lowers total cholesterol and low-density (harmful) cholesterol naturally
- Raises high-density (beneficial) cholesterol, which is an important marker for heart disease
- Lowers and stabilizes blood glucose levels by raising the metabolic rate and driving glucose out of the blood, into muscle cells
- Lowers insulin levels as glucose levels become more stable
- Increases aerobic capacity as the heart becomes stronger and oxygen utilization improves.
- Increases fat-burning by requiring more calories beyond the resting state
- Provides more stamina as heart and lung capacity increases
- Lessens fatigue
- Reduces blood-clotting tendency, a major risk factor for heart attack and stroke
- Increases sense of well being by increasing endorphin levels
- Reduces stress as endorphin levels are repeatedly elevated
- Periodic dilation of blood vessels makes them more flexible
- Regular lung expansion improves function
- Heart muscle becomes stronger in response to periodic exercise-induced stress

* Improves immune function, probably mimicking ancient stress responses
* It just feels good!

Finally, if you've ever put weight back on after having lost it, consider this. Ninety percent of individuals who lost weight and maintained that weight loss were regular exercisers. Of the people who regained the weight they had lost, only 34 percent were exercisers.

Is exercise dangerous?

It is dangerous not to exercise. When a heart attack occurs during exercise it is usually in a person who has not exercised regularly, especially those who exercise infrequently but intensely. Occasionally a young person is the victim of sudden death during physical activity, but most of those are individuals who have an undiagnosed heart abnormality. Some of these conditions can be detected during a medical examination.

Anyone can begin an exercise program, both aerobic and resistance type, at any age, provided that they undergo proper screening, instruction and supervision. There are specific effects of exercise that directly reduce the risk of sudden death from heart disease. Whatever problems may arise directly because of exercise, they are dwarfed by the immense benefits that we derive from it.

> *It's not exercise when your life depends on it.*

Five

The diabetes juggernaut

WHY DEVOTE AN entire chapter to diabetes? There are two reasons. First, type 2 diabetes mellitus is a clear example of what happens when genetics and lifestyle collide. Second, this form of diabetes has reached epidemic numbers in the United States affecting more than 18 million people. The disease increased by 38 percent from 1976 to 1994. Among persons below the age of 20 it is increasing even faster. Between 1982 and 1994 the incidence of type 2 diabetes increased ten-fold in children. The International Diabetes Federation estimates that the number of people around the globe with type 2 diabetes will double by the year 2030. This is surely an underestimate. It causes more deaths than motor vehicle accidents, according to the Centers for Disease Control, yet it is almost 100 percent preventable by means that we have, literally, at our fingertips.

Diabetes in a nutshell

Diabetes is an awesomely complex disease. Generations of brilliant researchers have been unable to completely unravel its mechanism or craft a cure. At the risk of becoming either too technical or too simplistic, I'll review it briefly, without getting into fat metabolism or the myriad of hormonal interactions that determine how our bodies process food for energy.

> **Where does the name *diabetes mellitus* come from?**
>
> Diabetes *comes from the Greek word for siphon and refers to the large and continuing outpouring of urine that afflicts patients.* Mellitus *is Latin for sweetened with honey. People in ancient times noticed that flies were attracted to the urine of diabetics. Early physicians diagnosed the disease by tasting the patient's urine.*

There are two kinds of diabetes, type 1 and type 2. Both are characterized by a high blood sugar (glucose), which is the primary source of energy for every cell in the body. In diabetes, glucose accumulates in the blood instead of entering cells. Directly and indirectly this results in progressive, severe abnormalities that affect every organ. Some are rapidly fatal and others take decades to develop. The exact mechanisms by which diabetes leads to kidney failure, blindness, narrowing of blood vessels, heart disease and stroke still elude us. The most likely mechanism is that excess glucose attaches itself to proteins and interferes with their function.

Type 1 used to be known as juvenile diabetes. Most victims are less than 30 years old but it occurs at all ages. These patients have a genetic predisposition to a defective immune process that destroys insulin-producing cells. They must take insulin by injection every day in order to survive. Lifestyle factors do not cause type 1 diabetes, although there are probably several environmental triggers that set the process in motion. (See Chapter Eight.)

Type 2 diabetes mellitus was once known as adult-onset diabetes, or non-insulin-dependent diabetes mellitus. Neither of those older terms is correct. The age of onset of type 2 diabetes is shifting downward, affecting 10 percent or more of persons between 20 and 30 years of age in some population groups. Pediatricians are discovering this form of the disease in patients as young as 10, sometimes earlier. In the later stages of the affliction some patients do require insulin, so the older term, non-insulin-dependent, is not appropriate, either.

Lack of exercise and inappropriate dietary intake in genetically susceptible persons are the main causes of type 2 diabetes. This sounds too simple, but it does not really contradict what we find in one of the leading textbooks of medicine, that type 2 diabetes "is a heterogeneous disorder with a complex etiology that develops in response to genetic and environmental influences." It's quite true that genetic factors have a very important role in the development of the disease. However, people with a very strong genetic susceptibility to type 2 diabetes do not fall victim to it unless and until they adopt a lifestyle that is discordant relative to their genetic endowment.

Type 1 diabetes certainly did exist in the Stone Age, and probably for millions of years before that. It causes death within a few weeks if it is not treated. Sam and Sal did not suffer from type 2 diabetes and neither do hunter-gatherers of today. An understanding of the pathway to type 2 diabetes will explain why.

The hallmark of diabetes is a chronic elevation of blood sugar. The calorie-sparse foods of less well developed societies (today's hunter-gatherers as well as those that lived in the millennia prior to the Agricultural Revolution) do not produce high levels of glucose in the blood, but the calorie-dense foods that form a large proportion of our modern diet do. Glucose that we do not immediately use for energy is stored in the form of glycogen. Almost all cells can store glycogen but most of it accumulates in the liver and muscles. When these stores of glycogen are filled to capacity the body converts the glucose that is left over to fat. This is a critical evolutionary survival mechanism, as I discussed in Chapter One. Some of us come from genetically fortunate stock: we have the ability to store fat very efficiently. But Nature never intended for us to carry it for the rest of our lives, or as in the case of morbidly obese individuals, to acquire several times as much fat as our lean body mass.

What is prediabetes?

Approximately 41 million persons in the United States have a fasting blood sugar of 100 or more, or have an abnormally high rise in blood sugar levels when they take a standard glucose (sugar) drink. Unfortunately, most of them don't know that they have this condition, called prediabetes. Yet almost all will find themselves with frank type 2 diabetes in the next 10 years unless they change their lifestyle.

This is an insidious transition to a devastating disease. It offers no warning signals and can smolder silently for years. The hallmark symptoms of type 2 diabetes, fatigue, increased thirst, frequent urination and deteriorating vision, are absent in prediabetes. All the while, though, a mild but persistent elevation of blood sugar is causing blood vessels to become narrower, lenses to become cloudier, blood pressure to rise gradually and cholesterol levels to creep upward. These changes are so subtle that nearly half of those with frank diabetes have already developed one or more complications of the disease at the time of diagnosis.

How successful we will be at slowing down the process depends on three simple measures: increased screening, increased physical activity and reasonable changes in our eating habits.

Being overweight is so common in type 2 diabetes that anyone over the age of 20 who is even a few pounds overweight should have a screening blood test at least every three years. Persons of certain high-risk racial groups (African-American, Asian-American, Latino, Pacific Islander, Native American), especially if there is a family history of diabetes, should obtain screening every year. Women who have had gestational diabetes (elevated blood sugar during pregnancy) have about a 50 percent chance of ultimately developing diabetes, especially if they are overweight.

If you are prediabetic you can lower your risk at least by half by simply getting more exercise on a regular basis. How much exercise? Thirty minutes a day of moderate physical activity, and it doesn't even have to be all at once. Three brisk 10-minute walks, if coupled with a diet that includes whole grains and more fruits and vegetables, lower the risk of progressing to type 2 diabetes by almost 60 percent.

What does insulin do?

Most people think of insulin as a medication for the treatment of diabetes. That is true for type 1 (insulin-dependent) diabetes mellitus. Persons with type 2 disease often have an excess of insulin, not a deficiency, at least in the earlier stages. The high but ineffective levels of insulin are responsible for some of the medical problems associated with type 2 diabetes.

Most of the carbohydrate we eat (and some of the protein) must be transformed into glucose before our bodies can make use of it. Insulin is a hormone that allows glucose to move from the bloodstream to the interior of cells that use it for energy to carry out the thousands of chemical reactions that make life and health possible.

Within limits, the higher our blood glucose, the more insulin we produce. If a person has frequent high levels of glucose as a result of taking in excess carbohydrates, cells will gradually become resistant to insulin. The body responds by producing higher and higher levels of insulin in order to drive glucose into cells. Insulin deficiency occurs when, at some point, the cells of the pancreas that produce this hormone become exhausted and fail to produce the hormone. When that occurs, the type 2 diabetic becomes like the type 1: he or she must take insulin daily by injection.

In the years between the diagnosis of diabetes and the exhaustion of the cells that produce insulin, various oral medications may lower glucose levels. There are several kinds of drugs for diabetes and they do not all work in the same way. Some increase the production of insulin; others improve the way the body uses glucose. One group slows the absorption of glucose from the intestine so that blood levels remain lower. Still another makes cells less resistant to insulin.

Sam and Sal didn't have access to foods that produced high blood glucose, so they didn't have persistently high levels of insulin. The insulin they produced performed its primary function of delivering glucose to the cells of the body. Insulin has one other role that helped Sam and Sal in their quest for survival: it prevents the release of stored fat. Tens of thousands of years later, it does the same in us. As I noted in Chapter Three, our bodies give up fat stores reluctantly, as if anticipating a future need for energy. Insulin is one of the factors responsible for this phenomenon and is thus another barrier to weight loss.

Insulin may contribute to two of the conditions that are associated with diabetes, namely, stroke and heart disease. It increases the body's production of cholesterol in the liver. The accumulation of cholesterol on the inner walls of blood vessels can lead to obstruction. If it occurs within the coronary arteries that supply the heart muscle the result is a heart attack. The same process in the arteries that supply the brain causes a stroke. Prolonged high levels of insulin have other damaging effects. It causes thickening of the muscle layer within arteries so that they become stiffer and narrower. It lowers HDL, known as good cholesterol, raises blood levels of triglycerides (a form of fat) and increases blood pressure, all of which are associated with an increased risk of stroke.

Elevated levels of insulin are also associated with a higher risk of colon and pancreatic cancer.

The genetic diabetic

Among Native Americans the Pimas are not the only tribe whose lifestyle changes have led to marked increases in diabetes and other noninfectious chronic diseases. Diabetes was once rare among all Native Americans. So was heart disease. Both of these diseases are now more common among Native Americans than among people of European descent. Obviously, their genes have not changed in the past century, but their lifestyle has.

The inhabitants of some Micronesian islands share the genetic predisposition of the Pimas toward obesity. Vegetables are easy to grow there and trees bend under the weight of fruit; fish thrive among the reefs and in the offshore depths. However, there is little incentive to harvest them. The United States gives monetary aid to many of these island governments and the jobs it provides require little physical effort. On other islands, phosphate mining has brought sustained wealth, even though the source of that wealth is now depleted. Fishing, growing vegetables and gathering fruit require manual labor, so islanders prefer to import processed, high-fat, calorie-dense foods. The bits of land on which they live are small and the inhabitants have little need for automobiles, but driving a car has status and walking does not. The result of all these factors is that among adults between the ages of 45 and 64, nearly 85 percent are obese, more than one-third have high blood pressure and more than a quarter have type 2 diabetes.

The Genetic Diabetic

An individual with the genetic tendency toward type 2 diabetes will more likely express that gene if:

* *his/her mother had overt type 2 diabetes*
* *mother was poorly nourished during pregnancy*
* *mother did not breastfeed*
* *he/she was obese in childhood*
* *he/she does not exercise*
* *he/she is obese as an adult*
* *he/she has a calorie-dense diet*

> ### What does the damage in diabetes?
>
> *The exact mechanism of how diabetes patients develop complications (kidney and nerve damage, heart disease, gangrene, cataracts, etc.) is as elusive as its primary cause. It seems to be due to damage of small blood vessels resulting from the interaction between the high levels of glucose and protein, a process called glycation.*

In almost every Native American, Alaskan or Polynesian group studied in the past quarter century, obesity and its fellow-traveler, type 2 diabetes, have been increasing dramatically, sometimes exponentially, wherever the Western lifestyle has penetrated. These problems still do not occur where the pre-contact lifestyle prevails. Physical activity is the linchpin. Mexican Pimas average 23 hours of occupational physical activity per week; Arizona Pimas average less than 5.

The Glycemic Index — easier than counting calories

All carbohydrate-containing foods contain glucose, but this vital packet of energy exists combined with other sugars or in long chains. In either case, Nature has equipped our bodies with enzymes capable of making glucose available for our cells' use. Depending on how quickly carbohydrates raise blood glucose after a meal, we classify them as low GI (low Glycemic Index) or high GI (high Glycemic Index). The index compares the rate at which carbohydrate-containing foods elevate the blood glucose compared with a reference food (white bread or glucose). In scientific terms it is the area under the curve. Low GI foods such as grapefruit, low-fat yogurt and lentil soup raise the blood glucose gradually. High GI foods (jellybeans, corn flakes, instant mashed potatoes) raise it rapidly and thereby call forth a greater outpouring of insulin. Frequent consumption of high GI foods produces repeated high levels of insulin and, eventually, insulin resistance.

We can modify the impact of high GI foods. First, we can simply eat them infrequently and in small amounts. That helps us to avoid the Martyr Mentality (Chapter Three) while still allowing us to enjoy our favorites from time to time. A second option is to combine them with low GI foods. That group includes most fruits and vegetables as well as some forms of pasta and rice.

> **Rating the Glycemic Index**
>
> *Low GI foods are those with a rating below 55. Those with a rating over 70 are high GI. The rest are intermediate. Don't be surprised if you find that various sources attribute different GI values to the same food item. These variations are relatively minor and change according to food source, method of preparation, etc. Appendix 3 contains a list of common foods and their glycemic index.*

There are some surprises on the list. Chocolate has a GI of only 44; ice cream is rated at 62. Parsnips are among the highest (97) and baked potato is 85. Keep in mind that the glycemic index is only one measure of nutritional value, and a narrow one at that. Not only are parsnips and baked potatoes generously endowed with healthful nutrients, but we usually eat them in combination with other, lower GI foods. That diminishes and prolongs the spike in glucose concentration. In spite of their relatively low GI, chocolate and ice cream are not exactly health foods. They are high in fat and mostly devoid of beneficial nutrients. White bread and whole wheat bread are almost identical (70 and 69, respectively) because both are finely milled. Stoneground whole wheat bread is somewhat lower, at 54. Table sugar has a lower GI than potatoes because it is composed of one molecule each of glucose and fructose. The liver must convert fructose to glucose, delaying its entry into the glucose pool. The starch in mashed or baked potatoes consists of long strings of glucose that begin to break down when they are heated. Enzymes in the saliva and intestines quickly split them into their glucose units for rapid entry into the bloodstream. That gives baked or boiled potatoes a high GI.

Low GI foods tend to satisfy the appetite at lower levels of calorie intake than high GI foods. Many have a high fiber content that produces an earlier sense of fullness. Compared with the standard diet for diabetics, one with high fiber significantly lowers blood glucose and insulin. Such a high fiber diet produces a decline in blood glucose similar to that which patients typically achieve when they take oral medication for that purpose.

Reported benefits of low GI diets include improved athletic performance, heightened mental alertness, less hunger, lower insulin levels and reduction in blood sugar.

There is bound to be some confusion between glycemic index and the complexity of carbohydrates. They are not directly related. Physicians have urged us in the past to avoid simple carbohydrates such as table sugar. They were thought to lead to obesity (and thus to type 2 diabetes) whereas complex carbohydrates like pasta, brown rice and potatoes would not. Most of the carbohydrate we consume consists of plant starch that exists in either straight chains or branched chains. Branching increases the surface area and provides more sites for cleavage by enzymes. Starches that are finely milled or partly degraded are subject to rapid breakdown into glucose. That gives them a high glycemic index. The germ layer that surrounds unmilled grains provides a temporary barrier to enzyme action so that these have a low glycemic index. Foods with high fiber content tend to be lower in glycemic index, but the correlation is not close. Some strains of starchy foods have a higher GI than others. Where foods are similar, different cooking methods will produce a different glycemic index.

The glycemic index may explain why obesity and type 2 diabetes continue to rise dramatically throughout the Western world in spite of a documented decrease in the consumption of fat. Low-fat diets have become more popular during the past 25 years but the fat has been replaced by carbohydrate. The added carbohydrate comes from processed foods with a high GI, not fruits and vegetables. We are witnessing a confluence of dietary changes drifting toward disaster. High GI foods contribute to persistent elevation of glucose and insulin; larger serving sizes in restaurants promote higher intake of calories overall (Chapter Six); a low-fiber diet bypasses one of the mechanisms that helps our bodies avoid type 2 diabetes; a reduction in antioxidant-rich fruits and vegetables limits protection from the harmful by-products of excess glucose. It is, indeed, a diabetes juggernaut that is bearing down on us.

Why Sam and Sal weren't diabetic

It takes a little imagination to visualize the kinds of fruits and vegetables that Sam and Sal ate. Unlike ours, which are large, juicy and sweet, theirs were small, fibrous and not very sweet. There were no foods made from wheat, rice or other grains. If they partook of any wild grain it came with its original complement of fiber and germ, which delayed digestion and lowered its glycemic index. By their nature, all these foods had a low glycemic index, did not raise blood glucose excessively and did not provoke a large insulin response. Aboriginal people in North America, Australia, Africa and India whose diet is high in low-GI legumes and other slow-release foods have a very low incidence of type 2 diabetes.

> **Didn't Stone Agers eat honey?**
>
> *Honey was a rare treat, not a staple. It is a seasonal crop and gathering it requires some effort. Vessels for storage and cooking were almost nonexistent for almost all of mankind's history, and so were the utensils necessary to remove honey from the comb.*

One of the most obvious differences between Sam and Sal's diet and ours is the amount of fiber and fat they consumed every day. Their fiber intake was approximately 15 times as high as ours; their saturated fat intake probably one-fifteenth as much. Wild game has only one-sixth as much saturated fat as contemporary meat.

They had no dairy products and no butter- or lard-containing pastries. These observations are of particular interest in light of a study that was carried out almost three decades ago in Australia. Aborigines with diabetes who reverted back to their traditional diet and lifestyle experienced considerable improvement in their blood sugar levels and other measurements in just a few weeks. An even faster response occurred among diabetic patients in a study at the University of Kentucky. When they ate a diet low in fat and high in fiber it took only two weeks for their cells to regain their sensitivity to insulin. This is consistent with other studies that show that the risk of diabetes decreases in men who replace refined grains with whole-grain foods.

Fructose, or fruit sugar, was a common carbohydrate in Sam and Sal's diet. As I noted above, their fruits were not as rich in this sugar as ours, but they had much more fiber, and because they were eaten fresh, they supplied more vitamins and antioxidants. Our diet contains much more fructose than Sam and Sal's because so many of our foods, especially fruit drinks, contain high-fructose corn syrup. This is a relatively inexpensive substance that is sweeter than glucose. The liver converts fructose to glucose but it does so slowly, giving fructose a fairly low glycemic index of 23.

> **Fructose: hard to avoid**
>
> *High-fructose corn syrup represents more than 40 percent of the sweeteners that manufacturers add to food products. Almost 100 percent of the added calorie-containing sweetener in soft drinks consists of high-fructose corn syrup. The next time you're at the supermarket, check the labels to see which foods do not have high-fructose corn syrup.*

Since 1970 the consumption of fructose has increased 10-fold, during which time obesity has nearly tripled. There are at least two reasons why high levels of fructose in our diet are playing a large part in the obesity epidemic. First, our bodies process fructose differently from glucose, so that it doesn't give us the feeling of full-ness that glucose does, especially when it's in liquid form. The result is that we take in too many calories. Second, large amounts of fructose in the diet lead to increased formation of the building blocks of fat.

> **Early complications**
>
> *There is a chilling aspect to type 2 diabetes in childhood. It appears that the complications that affect the heart, the eyes and the kidneys take less time to develop in persons who develop the disease in adolescence.*

Fructose does actually enhance the way in which we process glucose, and can improve the control of sugar in some persons with diabetes, but the amount is closer to what is found in natural fruit, not the excessive amounts that are now so prevalent in supersized drinks.

Complications of diabetes

Diabetes exacts an enormous price, not just in health but also in the quality of life. When I began my medical internship, one of the first patients to whom I was assigned was an African-American woman of middle years. The memory of her warm personality has never left me. Neither has the recollection of how her life was shattered and shortened by type 2 diabetes mellitus. She often recognized us by our footsteps, for she was blind; cataracts, glaucoma and retinal damage are typical effects of diabetes. I rarely saw her out of her hospital room; the disease led to amputation of one foot and chronic ulcers on the other. Her kidneys were failing, for even then, diabetes was one of the leading causes of that inexorably fatal condition. She died before I finished my internship, and long before she should have.

Ever wonder if your memory is slipping? We all do, of course, but it's another complication of type 2 diabetes. We've known for decades that diabetes causes narrowing of blood vessels everywhere in the body, including the brain, so it was no surprise that persons who have been diagnosed with diabetes show decreased memory and other mental abilities. But when apparently normal middle aged and elderly people were tested, those who had prediabetes did poorly. Further, those who handled glucose the least efficiently had the most severe impairment of memory. Their brain scans actually showed shrinkage of a particular part of the brain called the hippo-campus, which is involved with learning and memory.

Persons with insulin resistance are more likely to develop colon cancer and its precursors, known as colonic adenomas. Insulin may act as a growth factor, causing otherwise normal cells to prolif-erate and eventually become cancerous. In a study among Chinese men, there was an association between waist-hip ratio and cancer of the prostate. There is a connection between abdominal fat and elevated insulin levels. Follow-up studies seem to indicate that it is insulin, not obesity per se that is linked to prostate cancer.

Treatment doesn't compare with prevention

I cannot overemphasize the importance of preventing this disease with a healthy diet and lifelong physical activity, because there is no such thing as satisfactory treatment of type 2 diabetes. Damage to small blood vessels of the eyes, heart and kidneys occurs early, and about half of patients have an obvious complication by the time of diagnosis. After-the-fact lifestyle changes and medications can slow the progress of the disease, but not reverse it.

Most patients will not require insulin injections in the beginning, but may need to take a medication that will lower the need for insu-lin, or help it to work better. Some will be able to avoid medication by losing weight, adjusting their diet, and increasing physical activity. For most patients that is simply an impossible challenge, and they face inevitable hardships.

There are 5 different classes of oral drugs known as antihyper-glycemic agents for the treatment of type 2 diabetes, four of which may cause problems for persons with heart or kidney disease.

Nearly 100 patients died of liver failure, or required a liver transplant, before one drug was taken off the market.

Type 2 diabetes is often a part of a larger problem known as metabolic syndrome (sidebar), which adds to the complexity of treatment. Diabetic patients usually need medication for high blood pressure and elevated cholesterol.

Severe kidney damage is so common in this disease that the nation's dialysis centers can barely keep up with the demand. A news release from a manufacturer of dialysis units notes: "An aging population, coupled with diabetes-causing obesity, means cases of chronic kidney failure will continue to rise."

Type 2 diabetes has clearly become a growth industry in the twenty-first century. Before our youngest generation enters middle age there will be nearly one-half billion diabetics on this planet. Prevention is possible. Treatment is economically unsustainable.

The obesity factor

I stated earlier that type 2 diabetes is an awesomely complex disease. It takes years to develop and once established there is no real cure. Physicians struggle to slow down the course of the illness, to prevent its costly complications, and to provide its victims with a reasonable quality of life. Fortunately, avoidance of the disorder is simple, even among persons who have a strong family history of diabetes. What makes it difficult is the inability or unwillingness of the public to accept a high level of physical activity coupled with a low glycemic index, high fiber food intake. In other words, a Stone Age lifestyle.

Diabetes and obesity are clearly linked. In a study of Scandinavian patients, moderate obesity increased the risk of diabetes 10-fold; marked obesity increased it 30-fold. Observations among Native Americans and Pacific Islanders show a similar relationship between obesity and type 2 diabetes. Obesity is one of the major components of metabolic syndrome (Syndrome X), which includes impaired glucose and lipid (fat) metabolism, insulin resistance and hypertension. Even in children with type 2 diabetes, at least 85 percent are obese or overweight at the time of diagnosis. Among those who are not, obesity may have been masked by weight loss in the months prior to diagnosis.

Metabolic Syndrome*

Metabolic syndrome is an indicator of increased risk from type 2 diabetes as well as diseases of the heart and blood vessels. A person is defined as having metabolic syndrome if he or she meets 3 or more of the following criteria:

- *Abdominal obesity (waist circumference of >40 inches (102 cm.) in men, >34.5 inches (88 cm.) in women*
- *High blood pressure (= or >130/85)*
- *Elevated blood triglycerides (= or >150 mg/dL)*
- *Low HDL, "good" cholesterol (<40 mg/dL in men, <50 mg/dL in women)*
- *High fasting blood glucose (= or >110 mg/dL)*

* This has also been called Syndrome X and Insulin Resistance Syndrome

---

There is overwhelming evidence that overweight and obesity are associated with diabetes. Fat cells are not simply passive receptacles that become larger as excess glucose and fats pour into them. These *adipocytes* secrete several hormones whose function scientists are just beginning to unravel.

When blood glucose levels rise because of an excess of sugary or starchy foods, that overabundance calls forth an outpouring of insulin. When insulin disposes of the glucose, it often overshoots and sends the blood sugar lower than the optimal level. That triggers the sensation of hunger. This may seem like a vicious cycle, but it is consistent with the survival mechanism: accumulate as much fat as possible to prepare for the next downturn in the food supply. Sam and Sal, however, never had the prodigious and continuous sources of fat-producing foods that we have. Any accumulation of fat they had was modest. Obesity was not compatible with survival in their world.

It is not entirely accurate to say that obesity is simply the result of a high caloric intake. Sam and Sal and their contemporaries probably took in 3,000 or more calories per day, and Arctic explorers sometimes took in twice that much. Both groups expended the same number of calories that they took in so that they did not become obese. Whether or not they carried the genes for obesity didn't matter as long as they didn't take in more calories than they needed. In studies of obesity throughout the world, researchers point out that the determining factor is energy output, not energy input.

Exercise alone can help us to avoid obesity but it also takes a change in diet to avoid type 2 diabetes. As I noted in Chapter One, most of us become overweight by adding only an extra pound or two per year, a gain that we could easily avoid by burning just a few more calories a day. In order to avoid diabetes we also need to eliminate the insulin-stimulating spikes of blood sugar that we provoke when we eat refined carbohydrates — those with a high glycemic index. We can accomplish that by limiting our carbohydrates to those that we absorb slowly: fruits, vegetables, nuts and whole-grain breads and cereals.

In Chapter Six you'll find a simple, sensible strategy to accomplish that.

Six

Supermarket suicide and restaurant roulette

IN CHAPTER ONE I wrote that Sam and Sal, who lived about 50,000 years ago, were anatomically and physiologically almost identical to us. It was my intent to emphasize our physical similarities and to contrast our lifestyles. We can actually go back thousands of generations earlier, more than a million years perhaps, and find that biochemically the similarities persist. Those very distant ancestors, known as Homo erectus, walked upright, used tools and eventually controlled fire. Most importantly for our discussion, they ate the same kind of foods that Sam and Sal did: fruits, vegetables, roots, nuts, berries and wild game. Their body chemistry had evolved to process these foods, and until very recently there has never been evolutionary pressure for it to change. Although the roughly 15,000-year span since the beginning of the Agricultural Revolution seems like a very long time to us, it is not even an eye-blink within the cosmos. There has not been enough time since then for Homo sapiens to adapt to foods such as processed cereal grains and dairy products. It's even less likely for us to have adapted to the kinds of foods that have become available to us in the past few generations.

For reasons that I shall describe in Chapter Seven it's no longer possible to find foods such as those that nourished Sam and Sal.

Most of the wild predecessors of the fruits, nuts and vegetables we find today in supermarkets vanished as their habitats were replaced by farms, factories, houses and highways. They were very different from the large, juicy, sweet versions of the present century. The wild game in our fields and forests has no more fat than it did when Sam and Sal brought it down with sticks and stones, but now it contains pesticides and pollutants. Nutritionists advise that pregnant women limit their intake of swordfish, tuna and other fish because they represent the top of the marine food chain and have accumulated mercury and other toxins from below.

The U.S. Federal Drug Administration recommends that pregnant women avoid swordfish, shark, tilefish and king mackerel. The Environmental Working Group and the California Public Research Interest Group extend the pregnancy warning to tuna steaks, sea bass, Gulf Coast oysters, marlin, halibut, pike, walleye, white croaker and largemouth bass.

Those of us who live in the first world no longer face food shortages. Instead, we suffer from affluent malnutrition, and we have generously shared this maladaptive lifestyle with the poorest nations. In a brilliant article, Ellen Ruppel Shell has described New World Syndrome: A case study of how fatty Western plenty is taking a disastrous toll on people in developing countries. Her description of how Micronesia has descended from health and vigor to hypertension and diabetes in less than three generations reveals the consequences of bad choices, choices that are diametrically opposed to the Stone Age lifestyle.

During the Cold War, visitors from communist countries were amazed at the wide selection and abundant supply in our markets. That very abundance makes it possible for us to select the foods that will provide us with those nutrients that are compatible with our genetic endowment, or those that are not. By making the right choices we can avoid or postpone the so-called diseases of aging, maladies that are extremely rare among those who are aware of the

Secrets of the Stone Age. Persons who have attended my seminars tell me that the second most difficult lifestyle change is to change shopping habits. (The first is to start and then continue an exercise program.) My advice is the same for both challenges: do it, do it gradually, and do it sensibly.

Guidelines for sensible shopping

Advertising has a powerful influence on our habits. An ad for granola bars at a bus stop calls out, "Don't just stand there. Eat something!" It often wins out over common sense as our grocery cart rattles down the aisle. If you go food shopping when you're hungry you've lost the battle. If you always shop without a list the war is over. The awesome abundance in today's supermarket demands that we get in the habit of making sensible selections. We make these choices unconsciously in other areas of our lives every day. Who has to think before driving past the diesel pump at the service station? At the bookstore, does anyone stand and browse through titles in languages they don't understand? We can make rational, automatic rejection or selection of grocery store merchandise the same way — by habit.

The strategy of sensible shopping isn't complicated, and these guidelines provide a good starting point.

Ten tips for smarter shopping

Add more fruits and vegetables: Increasing our intake of fruits and vegetables is probably the most important change of all. Decades of research consistently show that a diet high in these foods lowers the risk of heart disease and cancer. Calorie for calorie, they are less expensive and more nourishing than anything else the market has to offer. They have adequate protein for anyone not engaged in intense physical activity. Vegetable fiber binds substances that lead to the formation of cholesterol and keeps them from being absorbed. Plant

---

Less lettuce, more spinach

Why is iceberg lettuce so popular? Probably because of its texture, what nutritionists refer to as mouth feel. If you insist on lettuce, make it the more nutritious Romaine variety. Fresh spinach is a smarter addition to salads and sandwiches. It has 3 times as much fiber, 5 times as much vitamin B2, B6 and folic acid, 7 times as much calcium and 28 times as much vitamin A (Pennington JAT, Bowes and Church's Food Values of Portions Commonly Used, 1998, Lippincott Williams and Wilkins publ., Philadelphia). *And it has a peppier flavor.*

(Caution: persons at risk of oxalate kidney stones should limit their intake of spinach.)

---

foods contain calcium, iron, vitamins and antioxidants. Together with nuts they provide the right kinds of fats. They fill us up quickly and satisfy our hunger.

If these were not reasons enough for increasing our vegetable intake, new research may have added another. Salicylic acid, otherwise known as aspirin, is present in small amounts in vegetables. Medical authorities agree that taking aspirin helps to prevent heart attacks and the most common type of stroke. The results are not yet conclusive, but it's possible that the heart-protective effect of a high vegetable intake may be related to its content of salicylic acid.

Select food items that have the right kind of fat, and keep it under 30 percent: The U.S. government guidelines suggest that we limit our fat intake to 30 percent of daily calories. Sam and Sal probably ate half that much, and we wouldn't feel deprived if we followed their example. Although it's possible to put together an extremely low fat diet, it wouldn't be very enjoyable and might be harmful. The

Ignore studies that claim that increasing daily fiber intake from less than 10 grams per day to 20 grams per day has no beneficial effect on health. That is true. But 20 grams per day really isn't very much, either. Sam and Sal took in about 150 grams per day, and even at the beginning of the twentieth century the average person ingested about 100 grams per day.

Nutrition Facts

Serving Size 7 Crackers (32g)
Servings Per Container About 8

Amount Per Serving

Calories 140　Calories from Fat 45

	% Daily Value
Total Fat 5g	8%
Saturated Fat 1g	5%
Polyunsaturated Fat 0g	
Monounsaturated Fat 1.5g	
Cholesterol 0mg	0%
Sodium 170mg	7%
Total Carbohydrate 22g	7%
Dietary Fiber 4g	15%
Sugars 0g	
Protein 3g	

Vitamin A 0%	Vitamin C 0%
Calcium 0%	Iron 6%
Phosphorus15%	Magnesium 10%

* Percent Daily Values are based on a 2,000 calorie diet. Your daily values may be higher or lower depending on your calorie needs:

	Calories:	2,000	2,500
Total Fat	Less than	65g	80g
Sat Fat	Less than	20g	25g
Cholesterol	Less than	300mg	300mg
Sodium	Less than	2,400mg	2,400mg
Total Carbohydrate		300g	375g
Dietary Fiber		25g	30g

sidebar shows a simple method for estimating the fat content of foods from the government-mandated nutrition label found on every package of prepared food. Precision isn't necessary and trying to achieve it will be a stumbling block to the practice of checking labels.

The quantity of fat is not the whole story, for there are some fats that we should always avoid, and some whose daily intake is critical to maintaining good health. A little reflection on Stone Age foods explains why.

Sam and Sal almost never had saturated fat, which is present primarily in domestic animal meats and their dairy by-products, and is virtually absent in wild game. Palm oil, coconuts and coconut oil also contain saturated fat, but coconuts didn't grow where Sam and Sal lived, and humans didn't produce vegetable oils until after the start of the Agricultural Revolution.

Trans fats are the most harmful. They prolong the shelf life of baked goods and other processed food, so manufacturers naturally began to use more and more of them. You won't find trans fats on product labels, but you can spot them by the term *partially hydrogenated.* Trans fats adversely affect

Total calories from fat should be less than 30 percent. Instead of mentally calculating the percentage of fat calories, just divide the total calories by 10 (e.g., 10 percent of 140 in the example = 14) and multiply by three (42). The label indicates 45 calories from fat. That's obviously more than 42, so if you want to keep your fat intake down, look for another product.

cholesterol metabolism and contribute to the development of heart disease, cancer and other chronic diseases.

Most vegetable oils also contain high levels of omega-6 fatty acids. There is an overabundance of these in the Western diet because they form a large component of commercial baked goods. Olive, flaxseed and canola oils are your best choices because they have relatively little of omega-6 precursors, and little saturated fat.

In their zeal to lower their fat intake, some people eliminate good fats as well. These are the monounsaturated and polyunsaturated fatty acids, and omega-3 fatty acids, about which I will say more in later chapters.

How does this translate into good shopping habits? In addition to keeping total fat calories below 30 percent for most foods, get in the habit of simply not buying foods likely to contain saturated fat and trans fat, and stocking up on foods that contain mono- and polyunsaturated fats.

Choose products that are whole-grain: Is all dark bread whole grain? Not at all. Food marketers know that most shoppers think that dark bread is whole wheat and don't read labels. That color may come from molasses, brown sugar or other ingredients. Only labels that list whole-wheat flour as the first ingredient really indicate whole-grain baked goods. Any other type of flour is white flour that has been stripped of its original nutrients and supplemented with various additives.

> *Coarsely ground flour spoils quickly because of the oils in it. When the milling process removes the oil-containing germ it will not become rancid. The end product, white flour, will keep indefinitely, because microbes, insects and vermin won't eat it.*

Pick the leaner cuts of meat: My father worked as a butcher for several years and frequently brought home well-marbled beef. He explained that it was laced with fat, which gave it extra flavor and thus made it the most desirable. The United States government confirmed this by labeling cuts of meat as prime, choice and grade in descending order of quality. Prime beef is that which contains the most fat. Good flavor does not equate to good nutrition, and experts now urge that we eat mostly leaner cuts of meat. Sam and Sal almost never had our equivalent of prime meat because animals in the wild are too active to accumulate large stores of fat unless they are preparing for hibernation.

Pass up foods whose label lists sugar as the first or second ingredient: Sugar is a nutritional void: no fiber, no protein, no vitamins, no minerals, no antioxidants. It serves only as a quick source of energy. Although I do not believe that sugar is toxic I feel that it is one of the leading contributors to the current worldwide epidemics of obesity and diabetes. In its various forms, sugar provides approximately 20 percent of the calories we consume every day. It is also the most difficult to identify, and hence to avoid, on food labels. A breakfast cereal, for example, may contain up to eight different forms of this carbohydrate. It may not be deliberate, but food manufacturers aren't likely to complain if customers can't recognize from the label that sugar is actually the first or second major ingredient in the product. It may be called maltose, corn syrup, high-fructose corn syrup, brown sugar, sucrose, dextrose, maltodextrin, malt syrup or honey. It's all sugar, though honey contains trace amounts of vitamins and antioxidants.

> *Don't be misled by "light" or "lite." It could refer to color, taste, salt, texture or calories. Some "light" bread is just sliced thinner. "Low cholesterol" does not mean fat-free. Look at serving sizes. It may mean one cookie. Read the labels!*

Don't shop when you're hungry: The most tantalizing foods are the ones with lots of sugar or fat, and you might eat a few cookies before you even get out of the store.

These dense-calorie foods are usually the most expensive. You'll save a few dollars every week by shopping when you have little or no desire for them.

Don't shop for groceries with the kids: If they do have to come along, make sure that they're well fed and well rested. If you have to pacify them while you're shopping you'll probably reach for some sugary snack.

Stay away from the lady who's handing out free samples: These are usually fried or fatty, or they contain cheese or processed meat. They also have a tempting, appetizing aroma that is meant to draw you to that area of the store. Promotional foods tend to be expensive and have a high profit margin.

Don't just look at fat on the label: No fat, low fat, fat free or reduced fat foods might be honestly labeled, but they may contain lots of calories from sugar. Low fat doesn't mean low calorie so that you can have two servings.

Don't shop with a friend: If they put something tempting but fattening in their cart you might do the same. If you do need a companion when you go to the supermarket, pick a skinny one.

Dining in

By the time Sam and Sal appeared on earth, man had been using fire for several hundred thousand years. For most of that time there were no cooking utensils, as we know them. They cooked meat over an open flame, or they may have steamed vegetables in a pit, as in a Hawaiian luau or Cape Cod clambake. They probably ate their fruits and most vegetables raw. There were no baked goods because harvesting and processing wild grain involves the use of specialized tools for grinding and heating. This is the culinary lifestyle that molded our evolutionary legacy.

The first step toward a healthy home cuisine is to stop frying, especially deep-frying. Not only are cooking oils and fats high in calories, but when heated they undergo changes that are a further detriment to health. In *Eating Well for Optimum Health* (Alfred A. Knopf, publ., New York, 2000, p. 90), Dr. Andrew Weil discusses the hazards of heated vegetable oils. At high temperatures some fats produce toxic substances that injure the inner lining of blood vessels, reducing blood flow. Replace your frying recipes with those that use sautéing instead. You can use a minimum of oil, or even substitute with water, wine, chicken broth, Worcestershire sauce or fruit juice. Nonstick utensils and vegetable sprays have made it easier to eliminate traditional fried foods. An added benefit is the reduced fire hazard when we eliminate frying.

Use a rack when you roast meats so that you can easily discard the fat that drips into the pan below, or use it for gravy. Then use a pour-from-the-bottom gravy pitcher so that less fat is poured onto your plate.

You can easily lower the fat content of soups and gravies. Leave them in the refrigerator overnight and skim off most of the congealed fat.

It's easy to trim away excess fat before you cook meat, but if you start with leaner cuts such as London broil or top round you'll save yourself even that inconvenience.

Take advantage of the lower fat content of turkey and use it as a replacement for beef in some of your favorite recipes such as meat loaf, hamburgers, tacos, lasagna, etc.

For dishes like soups, stews and burritos, replace the meat with beans. You'll still get lots of protein, but without saturated fat.

Dairy products offer a good example of how you can gradually lower the fat content of your diet. If your family enjoys whole (3 percent) milk, buy 2 percent for a month or so, then 1 percent, then skim. You can do the same with cheese, but there are so many varieties and brands on the market that you'll need to experiment a little. Some low-fat cheeses are virtually indistinguishable from regular, but others will test your determination as well as your palate.

Fruits, especially apples and bananas, are among the best "subs" in your kitchen. Get in the apple habit by adding them to salads, cereal, desserts, tuna and chicken casseroles, meat loaf and your personal favorite recipes. Applesauce or bananas can replace up to half the butter or shortening in your baking recipes. (Hint: replace only about ¼ of the butter or shortening until you learn what pleases your palate.) Add some banana to your next meat loaf.

Other substitutions include using nonfat yogurt in place of mayonnaise, which is 90 percent fat, in tuna salad. (Start with tuna packed in water, not in oil.) For sandwiches, use less mayo and more mustard.

Don't carry substitution too far. The concern over cholesterol has encouraged many people to abandon eggs, or to cook with egg substitutes. We forget that Sam and Sal were very good at finding eggs, just like their earliest savannah-dwelling forebears and modern hunter-gatherers. Our body chemistry can accommodate this food source quite well. Unless you eat eggs just about every day there is no reason to eat fewer of them. There are more than 200 milligrams of cholesterol in an egg, but eating one or two a few times a week will not have nearly the effect on your blood cholesterol as "egg partners": bacon, sausage, ham and butter. These are high in saturated fats and have a much greater role than eggs in raising your cholesterol. When you eliminate eggs you remove a healthy source of essential fatty acids, protein, folic acid, vitamins D and E and several B vitamins. If you are still worried, I suggest that you discard two yolks for every three eggs you use. You'll barely notice the difference in flavor or color.

When you reduce fat and salt, some of your favorite dishes will seem a little bland, but this offers a great opportunity to get to know your spice rack better. We usually assume that spices and condiments were developed to make food tastier. Another reason that the use of spices became so widespread was food spoilage. Until refrigeration came into wide use we relied on stored ice, which was obviously available only to the wealthy, and only where it was practical. An adept cook could sometimes salvage foods that were just a little "off" by disguising early deterioration with well-chosen spices. If you wonder about food poisoning, remember that it is due to certain microorganisms and not all spoiled food is dangerous. In fact, ancient Romans savored garum, also known as liquamen, a fermented fish sauce. Eskimos still savor mikiyak, a mixture of fish, seal meat and whale blubber. They let it ferment in a large container until bubbles form on the top.

> ### The Feast Day Concept
>
> *By now you may be lamenting the loss of your favorite foods. My answer is the Feast Day concept: eat whatever you'd like on holidays such as Thanksgiving, Christmas, your birthday, etc. You might find a reason to feast as often as once a month, but if it's much more often, the consequences are obvious.*

Pass (by) the salt, please

Sam and Sal probably took in about 700 milligrams of sodium a day. They were omnivores, eating both animal and plant foods, and didn't have to seek out salt deposits, as many plant-eaters do.

A high intake of sodium isn't the only cause of high blood pressure, but it certainly is a major one, especially in certain population groups. African hunter-gatherers eat about 600 milligrams of sodium a day, about as much as Sam and Sal did, and they have virtually no hypertension. Among their genetically identical counterparts in the United States, salt intake is about 4 times higher, and hypertension is a leading cause of death.

Physicians counsel patients with hypertension and heart failure to follow a low-sodium diet, about 1,000 milligrams daily. For anyone who has ever tried it, it seems bland and unappetizing, but that's still more sodium than our body chemistry is designed for. That's because it's remarkably easy to acquire a preference for a much higher salt intake. One 8-ounce serving of tomato juice contains more than 800 milligrams; a single slice of cheese pizza has almost as much; a tablespoon of soy sauce has more than 1,200 milligrams.

If you automatically reach for the saltshaker before you even take the first bite of dinner, you're probably getting a lot more sodium than your body needs. If you can resist the temptation to salt your food, avoid dishes that are obviously highly salted, such as cheese and processed meats, and become aware of nutrition labels when you shop, you can gradually lower your intake to more healthy levels. Aim for 2,400 milligrams a day or less. It isn't necessary to get down to hunter-gatherer levels in order to gain major health benefits. You'll probably lose your taste preference for salty foods within just a few weeks. In a couple of months even potato chips may seem too salty for you.

> Try these accentuators in place of table salt: black and red pepper, jalapeno peppers, onions, garlic, horseradish, curry, ginger, Worcestershire and A-1 sauces, Tabasco, balsamic vinegar.

Can you really make kale and Brussels sprouts taste good?

Kids hate 'em, and adults don't think much of them either. There must be some cosmic reason why vegetables that are so well endowed with nutrients are so unappealing to so many people! Kale, broccoli, beets, cabbage, Brussels sprouts and spinach are loaded with vitamins and antioxidants, but they rank far below such favorites as corn, carrots and potatoes.

The cruciferous vegetables, broccoli, cabbage and Brussels sprouts, contain sulphoraphane and isothiocyanates, agents that protect us against cancer. Other factors lower cholesterol and may reduce the risk of autoimmune diseases such as lupus. There ought to be some way to make them more likeable — and there are.

Let's face it. This is not a colorful group. No matter how rich they may be in calcium, vitamins A, C and K, lutein and other nutrients, they just aren't very appealing. Here are some tips that will make them look better and taste better, but will not require lots of extra time to prepare.

Get 'em while they're young. Brussels sprouts, green beans and beets become more bitter and woody when they mature and lima beans develop a mealy texture. You'll find that the younger, smaller ones cook faster, are more tender and have a snappier, sweeter flavor.

Overcooking is a culinary crime. When cabbage and broccoli are overcooked they release odor-bearing sulfur compounds from those cancer-fighting sulphoraphanes and isothiocyanates that I described earlier. Asparagus, beets and green beans don't have an odor, but boiling diminishes their bright color as well as their nutrient value. You can preserve both qualities by steaming them lightly. Sautéing keeps bell peppers, asparagus and mushrooms with near-fresh crispness.

No fancy recipes needed. Just sprinkle slivered or chopped almonds, cashews, walnuts, or whole pine nuts on any kind of vegetables. Nuts provide healthy fats, minerals and protein. Powder some Parmesan cheese on kale, broccoli or lima beans. Add a little powdered clove to beets. A pinch of caraway seeds will soften the remaining bitterness of Brussels sprouts. Mint, marjoram and cumin add zing to squash, peas and green beans.

Experiment a little. Tired of boiled spinach? I was, so I decided to add a little of this and a little of that from the spice rack. It became a family tradition: Dad's Spinach Surprise. I tried various combinations of caraway seed, Italian seasoning, allspice, sage, thyme, etc. Everybody's favorite was curry powder. As long as you're not heavy-handed it's hard to go wrong, and it's always different.

Uncommon combinations. Add lemon pepper, maple syrup or nutmeg to your broccoli, cabbage or Brussels sprouts recipe.

Try sample-size servings. A traditional dinner consists of one serving of meat or fish, one serving of pasta, potatoes or rice, and one serving of cooked vegetable. There's no rule that says that only one vegetable belongs on the plate, but even restaurants follow that dictum. The low-carb mentality that has gripped the nation in the past few years gives us the perfect opportunity to break the bonds of tradition as many people are looking for alternatives to carbohydrate-rich meals. These ugly ducklings of the vegetable world, broccoli, kale, cabbage, Brussels sprouts, etc., have such a low GI (page 98) that most Glycemic Index tables do not even list them, or lump them under a single category at the bottom of the chart! Yet, all of Sam and Sal's carbohydrate came from low-GI vegetables, roots and fruits.

Instead of the usual mashed potatoes or pasta, why not put three or even four small helpings of different vegetables on the plate? The variety will add to the interest. Children, especially, when confronted with little more than a dollop of previously disdained foods, might be more willing to try them.

Make yours a soup kitchen. You may have wondered where the rhyme "Peas porridge hot, peas porridge cold, peas porridge in the pot nine days old" came from. It refers to the kettle in medieval kitchens, which received every meal's leftovers. Our grandmothers knew that the ultimate disguise for leftovers, or for things like okra, is soup. You can make it one of the most nutritious elements of your family menu by including vegetables that most people would avoid as a stand-alone serving. The average cook can easily hide kale, summer squash, even broccoli, in a well-flavored soup.

Dress up your salads. They won't call it rabbit food if you take advantage of what is probably already in your kitchen. Chunks of apple, pear or pineapple take only a minute or two to prepare, and mandarin oranges come right out of the can. Use artichoke hearts, dried currants or chopped olive (singly, not in combination) to make them taste different every time. Mince a few dried plums (the politically correct term for prunes) to add to a bowl of salad greens.

Desserts

Desserts are the downfall of dieters. Don't give them up; give them class. Sorbets and sherbets, frozen juice bars and fat-free puddings have little or no fat. They do, however, con-

Enjoy Italian-style dessert: a small scoop of sorbet (about one table-spoonful) topped with fresh fruit. About one-half teaspoon of creme de menthe or creme de cassis gives it a piquant elegance.

tain sugar, so don't serve them every day. Angel food cake has less than half the calories of most desserts, and almost no fat. (No wonder they call it angel food.)

Safe Snacks

We all get cravings and urges. The secret is to only have on hand calorie-sparse, filling foods. Here are some examples:

- *apples or other favorite fruit, either fresh or dried**
- *baby carrots*
- *fat free frozen yogurt*
- *tea — regular and herbal*
- *fat free hot cocoa mix*
- *peanut butter*
- *fruit preserves with no added sugar*
- *protein bar*
- *walnuts or almonds*

* Limit dried fruit to 3 or 4 pieces. They are more calorie-dense than the other snacks on the list.

Why not water?

Water is the most underappreciated beverage to which we have access. For almost all of the past few million years, the only beverage available to humans besides water was breastmilk. After infancy, Sam and Sal had virtually nothing else to drink. Water that comes from a safe source is ideal for humans. Our body chemistry is perfectly adapted to it. It's not only a thirst-quencher but often satisfies the appetite as well. What we occasionally feel as hunger is actually thirst, and a glass of cool water will sometimes relieve hunger pangs.

We take for granted the scores of fluid foods in our homes, supermarkets and workplaces. None of these existed before the Agricultural Revolution. Beer and wine awaited the cultivation of grain and grapes. Fruit juice is a modern invention and the fruit drinks that masquerade as juice are a culinary crime. Their true juice content may be 10 percent or less, and almost all the calories they contain come from various forms of sugar. Instead of making juice, Sam and Sal ate fruit and drank water. That meant they got carbohydrates, vitamins, minerals, antioxidants, fiber and fluid and no preservatives.

How much water is enough?

Six to eight glasses a day? Twelve glasses a day? One ounce for each 2 pounds of body weight? Your body's water requirements vary greatly depending on ambient temperature, humidity, your work and exercise pattern, the foods you eat, etc. No numerical formula fits everyone, but most of us should drink at least 60 ounces a day. The best gauge is the color of your urine. If it's dark and pungent, you're not getting enough fluid. The color should always be light yellow or straw-colored in order to maintain proper fluid balance and to avoid kidney stones.
When you exercise moderately in hot conditions, aim for about one pint an hour.

Could some of the recent rise in obesity be due to an increase in the intake of liquid food? Some nutrition experts think so. They note that fat intake has been decreasing for the past couple of decades, but carbohydrate intake, largely in the form of soft drinks, has gone up. Between the early 1980s and the mid-1990s, our soft drink intake increased by almost one-half, and our intake of juice rose by 22 percent.

Energy derived from liquids doesn't satisfy our hunger, so that we tend to take in more calories than if that energy came from solid food. Scientists aren't sure why; several mechanisms are involved. The act of chewing (mastication) sends a message to the brain that limits our hunger. We don't have to chew liquids, of course, so we miss that satiety signal. Eating solid food also starts our digestive juices flowing; liquids don't do that. Insulin plays a role in limiting hunger, but the response after a fluid meal isn't as strong as it is after a solid meal. The net result is that fluid calories are add-ons that add weight.

Is plain water too bland for you? Enhance it without adding many calories by keeping a tray of cranberry juice ice cubes handy. It takes just a moment to drop one into your glass. Cut a lemon or lime into wedges and store these right alongside the water pitcher in the refrigerator. For variety you can keep a few mint leaves in the same container. Crush the leaves slightly before placing them in the glass.

> **Does everybody need milk?**
>
> *Even though cow's milk is not an ideal food (except for baby cows) it does provide a source of calcium, protein and vitamin D. The disadvantages of whole cow's milk, excess fat, allergy-inducing protein and sometimes-indigestible sugar (lactose), do not yet outweigh its benefits for most of us. The story is not over, however. Contaminants such as hormones, antibiotics and other chemicals may yet tip the balance to make cow's milk a poor food choice in the future.*

Dining out

Americans eat 40 percent of their meals outside the home. The competition for this business is fierce, and has led to an insidiously unhealthy tactic: an escalation of larger servings. This marketing

Between 1957 and 1997:

- *The average muffin grew from 1.5 oz. to 8 oz. (1/2 pound).*
- *Fast food hamburgers went from less than 2 oz. to 6 oz.*
- *The 8-oz. soft drink reached 32 to 64 oz.*
- *Movie popcorn followed the size trend of the screen, and went from a 3-cup portion to 16 cups.*

phenomenon would be a boon to consumers if they ate appropriate portions of these mega-meals and put the rest in a take-home container for the next day. But that's not happening; most people eat whatever they are served.

Most of the cost of a restaurant meal comes from overhead, including labor. Actual food costs are only 25 percent, or less, of the total so that restaurant managers can make servings seductively larger for a small increase in price. In the middle of the last century a portion of steak consisted of about 4 ounces and 260 calories. At a well-known restaurant chain it weighs 14 ounces and yields more than 1,200 calories. A walk-in-waddle-out restaurant in Texas serves a 72-ounce steak. The standard serving of pasta at a popular chain of Italian restaurants contains 25 ounces, more than 1½ pounds.

It's a rare restaurant that doesn't offer alcoholic beverages. This is excellent market-

Do they serve too-large portions at your favorite restaurant? Before you begin the entree, divide it into two or three portions and eat only one. Take the rest home.

If you wait until you're partly through with your meal it's easier to eat it all.

ing strategy for two reasons. First, the profit on wine, beer and mixed drinks is very high. What the customer pays for two glasses of wine is usually more than the restaurant pays for the entire bottle. Unless a patron asks for a mixed drink containing a specific brand of whiskey, the bartender's choice is the bottle with the lowest cost.

Second, alcohol serves as an aperitif, the French word for appetizer. While you drink an alcoholic beverage you are more likely to order the fried chicken wings or zucchini. (Have you ever considered that these items comprise two of the least expensive raw materials in the entire restaurant? Yet you'll usually pay $3–5 for them.) Alcohol taken before a meal stimulates food intake whereas simple fruit juice does not. When you have juice, soup or salad at the start of a meal you'll reach a feeling of fullness sooner, so that you'll be less likely to order dessert.

The first item the waiter places on the table is usually the bread-basket, with the customary half-dozen packets of butter. (What does that tell you about the real cost of butter?) As I noted in Chapter Five, The Diabetes Juggernaut, bread products made from refined flour have a high glycemic index (GI) and produce not only a spike in blood sugar, but also a spike in insulin. Butter is almost pure saturated fat, and insulin drives fat from the bloodstream into fat cells.

> A person who eats a single extra pat of butter a day and does not expend the equivalent amount of energy will gain eight pounds a year.

Could there be a more efficient mechanism for obesity? I suggest that you continue to enjoy bread or rolls before dinner, but ask for whole-wheat products. If you do need to put something on your bread or roll, ask for some olive oil with balsamic vinegar, and send the butter back.

If a green salad is part of the dinner package, take it. Although iceberg lettuce is almost a nutritional void, except for folic acid, at least it has no fat and contributes to satiety. Most salad dressings are high in fat. Ask for your favorite one on the side and dip your fork into it with each mouthful instead of pouring it over the top of the salad. You'll enjoy all the flavor and a fraction of the fat calories.

We can avoid fried foods at home and it's even more important to pass them by when eating out. The oil used in deep-frying is seldom the healthiest grade and prolonged heat promotes oxidation and the formation of artery-damaging toxic compounds. If you order sautéed foods you can request that oil be used sparingly or not at all. Water, wine or other ingredients for sautéing are not a challenge to a competent chef.

Fatty red flags

There are no nutrition labels on restaurant menus, but here are some descriptive terms that indicate a high fat content: creamed, crispy, breaded, a la king, croquettes, carbonara, parmigiana, meuniere, tempura, fritters, frito, Alfredo, au gratin, au beurre, batter-dipped, bearnaise, hollandaise and Newburg. (List quoted directly from Wellness Made Easy; 365 Tips for Better Health, *University of California at Berkeley Wellness Letter, 1995, Health Letter Associates.)*

Don't be reluctant to ask for minor changes in preparation of your food choice, especially in a restaurant that you visit fairly often. You can have your meat entrée with the fat trimmed off beforehand, a smaller baked potato, extra vegetables in place of potatoes au gratin, and any reasonable but healthful variation on the menu. Remember that your patronage and the tip put you in control.

Smorgasbord: the Swedish word for "all you can eat"[1]

The American penchant for trying to squeeze a little more value from a dollar is evident in the buffet-type restaurant, sometimes called a smorgasbord. Older persons on fixed incomes and families on tight budgets push overloaded trays of food along silvery tracks toward the cashier. Just like the supermarket, there are good choices and bad choices.

The first group of foods consists of the salads: tong salads and spoon salads. Tong salads consist of leafy, green and yellow vegetables that you pick up with tongs. A plateful has few calories and considerable bulk. It's intended to blunt your appetite for the more

---

[1] Not really. The word actually means bread and butter table (*Thorndike-Barnhart Comprehensive Desk Dictionary*, 1962 Doubleday, New York). (Alternative meaning: sandwich table, *Encyclopedia Americana* 2001, Grolier, Danbury CT.)

expensive entrees. Salads that you pick up with a spoon are those made with pasta, potatoes and creamy dressings. A plateful of this will likely provide you with all the calories you need for the day. Small crocks of salad dressing await you at the end of this section.

The first rules of all-you-can-eat dining are: take the tong salads, go easy on the spoon salads and put the dressing on the side of the plate, not all over the contents.

The seafood entrees are usually boiled, broiled or fried. The first two are fine. I've already discussed why you should avoid deep-fried foods. Meats are often served in thick sauces. You should approach these as if they are condiments, not main courses. That is, take a normal serving, which is approximately the size of your palm, not including the fingers.

Most people take dessert when they first enter the serving line and are likely to put two or three on the tray. After all, they're usually the most attractive items in the food line, especially when you're hungry. They are also cheap. Why do you think the management puts them up front? Discipline yourself to eat your regular meal slowly and go back later for dessert. If three or four really do look irresistible, take them back to your table where you can share them with others.

> Your body has an appestat designed to limit your food intake to what you need. When the stomach fills, it sends a signal to the brain to limit the appetite. It takes about 20 minutes to reach that point for most people. Your mother was right when she told you to chew your food completely and eat slowly. Well-designed research studies back her up.

Eating ethnoid

Ethnoid is a more fitting term than ethnic. Emigrants and visitors from other countries have told me that the international foods they find here are often very different from the dishes available in their homeland. From my own experience I know that this is true. In spite of that we have a wonderful selection of foreign restaurants from which to choose. Their menus are conspicuously different from each other and provide pleasant variety. In countries considerably smaller than the United States there is a tremendous variation from region to region, so it's not easy to define a truly national cuisine. Italian food is a good example. The typical menu in northern Italy has more meat and dairy products than one in the south. This richness gradient matches the coronary gradient. The incidence of heart disease among Italians is higher in the north.

Italian

So many Italian dishes have become commonplace in the United States that most items on this menu are part of our home cuisine. Tomato sauce, olive oil and garlic are some of the healthiest ingredients of Italian cooking. Although less conspicuous in the United States than in Italy, fish and lots of fresh vegetables are part of the genuine Italian diet. The American-Italian restaurant menu is much higher than the so-called Mediterranean Diet in meat, fat, cholesterol and sodium.

Italians enjoy a variety of cheeses but in my travels there it never seemed to dominate as it does in the United States. This is especially true of pizza, on which cheese is used sparingly in Italy. Even though no-cheese pizza seems like an oxymoron, by adding extra tomato and a variety of vegetables (broccoli, sweet pepper, mushrooms, eggplant, olives, onions) it becomes a tasty, filling and healthy dish. On the other hand, pepperoni,

> Cioppino is one of the healthiest items on the Italian menu. The primary ingredients, fish, shellfish, shrimp and tomatoes, make it an abundant source of antioxidants (vitamin C, lycopene), omega-3 fatty acids, potassium, vitamin B12, iron and magnesium.

sausage, and Canadian bacon quickly convert it into something entirely different.

Good choices include cacciatore dishes and cioppino, minestrone, and red clam and wine sauces. Most lasagna and manicotti recipes are high in fat calories; so are Alfredo and white clam sauces. Skip the garlic bread.

In Italy, off the tourist track, desserts consist only of fruit. Tiramisu and multiple-layer cakes are holiday treats.

Mexican

A generation or two ago only Southwesterners were familiar with these foods. You'll find them now in the remotest corner of the United States. Inexpensive, filling and flavorful, Mexican dishes go far beyond tacos, tostadas, burritos and enchiladas. North American versions tend to be high in fatty meats (pork and beef) but chicken and fish are more representative of many areas in Mexico. Beans are healthy ingredients of Mexican dishes, but beans refried in lard are not. Chorizos, crispy tacos, quesadillas, flautas, chimichangas and nachos are high in fat; enjoy them in small quantities.

Bean burritos and other dishes made with unfried corn tortillas are good choices. Gazpacho and ceviche have plenty of vegetables.

Chinese

It seems odd that we should characterize as one entity a country that spans 4,000 miles and 6 time zones, and represents a fifth of the world's population. Granted that what we accept as Chinese food is not what the average person eats in China (they eat very little meat), its uniqueness and emphasis on steamed vegetables, chicken and seafood place it in good company. Bok choy, bean sprouts, tofu and mushrooms add various nutrients. There are several high-fat fried foods on the Chinese menu such as sweet and sour pork, egg rolls and spring rolls, and "crispy" anything. If you enjoy fried rice, mix it with plain white rice in order to lower the fat content. Limit spare ribs, duck and egg foo yong to feast days.

Chopsticks are a challenging change from Western flatware. The disposable ones we use in Asian restaurants are a cost-effective alternative to forks, which are relatively expensive and must be cleaned after every use. Unless you are very experienced you'll eat more slowly with chopsticks, so you'll tend to eat less.

Japanese

It's no surprise that the Japanese have one of the highest life expectancies in the world, and women in Japan have the lowest rate of breast cancer. Their diet emphasizes soy, seafood and vegetables, and little red meat. They do, however, have a very high salt intake. Avoid dishes such as tempura, which is deep-fried. Good choices include sushi, sashimi, yakisoba and yakimono dishes. Teriyaki dishes tend to be salty.

Oy! Soy!

Few condiments match the sodium content of soy sauce. Only 2 tablespoons contain 2,454 milligrams. That's more than the Daily Value (2,400 milligrams)

Indian

Not many Americans are familiar with Indian food. Like the Chinese cuisine, it varies widely according to geographic differences, and doesn't represent what most people in that country eat. It's best to ask your server if the menu doesn't describe the ingredients and methods of preparation. Some dishes are prepared with coconut oil, some with ghee (clarified butter).

French

In discussing food, the words rich and French are almost synonymous. In the everyday life of the Frenchman they are not. The better establishments in France, as well as in the United States, showcase the exquisite sauces and sophisticated recipes that have become famous. Both here and in France I have observed that those wonderful sauces adorn only small portions of fish, fowl or beef. Steamed or poached, prepared in vegetable, fruit or wine sauces, fish and fowl contain relatively small amounts of fat. A few typical dishes are high in fat, including duck and goose, escargot in butter, foods prepared with cream sauces, and croissants.

French desserts are dazzlingly decadent. They are usually small, even dainty, so that indulging in them doesn't seem irresponsibly unhealthy. Still, save them for feast days.

The French Paradox: If foods in France are so rich, why do the people who live there have a lower rate of heart disease than Americans? Scientists refer to this as the French Paradox. Is it the wine? Is it their genes? Is it real?

Reporting methods might account for some of the difference, but not all. Food portions are smaller there. In Paris, France, the size of a steak is 6 ounces; in Paris, Texas, it's 16 ounces. The French eat less meat, and the rich sauces of Parisian restaurants are not part of their daily fare. Their biggest meal is at midday; ours is in the evening, which is more likely to add to our excess weight. Not only do the French eat more vegetables and fruits than other Europeans, many families grow their own. Fresh produce is available to them for much of the year, and is three times as varied as that in the United States. The French are less mechanized and more active than Americans, and regular physical activity is clearly protective against coronary artery disease.

The French tend not to be binge-drinkers even though their consumption of alcohol, mostly in the form of wine, is relatively high compared to other Europeans. The observation that the alcohol intake of French women is approximately one-third of that for men may contribute to the lower incidence of heart disease.

The French Paradox may be sinking into history. As they, and people all over the globe, adopt our eating patterns and fast food lifestyle, their rates of obesity, heart disease, stroke and diabetes are rising.

Greek

The wide range of ingredients and cooking methods in Greek recipes reflects the variety in the topography and demographic history there. The basic ingredients of the mainland and the islands are similar to those of the Stone Age: fruits, vegetables, nuts, seeds and fish. The Americanized version of Greek food includes more generous servings of cheese and meat. Even moussaka is similar to our version of Italian lasagna, with layers of eggplant, meat and cheese covered with a white sauce.

The traditional diet of Greece is one of the world's healthiest, and studies done on the island of Crete (see Chapter Nine) are, belatedly, contributing to a new appreciation of the true Mediterranean diet.

In summary, truly ethnic food is difficult to find in the United States. In all the countries I mentioned, meat is relatively scarce except among wealthier families. Most household fare tends toward vegetarianism. American versions of ethnic restaurants may be exotic in their atmosphere, but they serve what sells, namely, dishes that contain more meat, fat, sugar and salt than their alleged equivalents in the home country.

When you're a guest

Breaking bread together has been a way of establishing close bonds of friendship for millennia. There is something very special about dining at a friend's house. Bringing the boss home for dinner is probably an older custom than we think. When we are guests we might encounter foods that we would ordinarily avoid because they have too much fat or sugar. I suggest that you make the hostess happy: unless you have a food allergy or intolerance, one unhealthy meal won't undermine your well-being. Consider it a Feast Day. Above all, don't make an issue of being on a diet, even if you are.

That doesn't mean that you have to eat every single particle of food on your plate. It's easy if it's a buffet. Use the strategy I described above for all-you-can-eat restaurants. Take small portions of what looks best and go back only for what you like. Start with fruit if it's available and stay away from salads that are served with a spoon. Take only one dessert at a time. Move away from the buffet table while you're eating. Drink more water than wine.

Resist the invitation for seconds, even if the hostess claims it will otherwise go to waste. Of course it will go to waste; it will go to *your* waist.

How to enjoy a party

Party fare is invariably high-fat, high-sugar and high salt, which will encourage you to drink more. If there's a vegetable tray you'll usually find a high-fat dip in the middle of it. Start with the veggies anyway, and dip sparingly. Take the edge off your appetite before the hors d'oeuvres tray makes its way to you. We often pluck them from a passing tray while we're in the middle of conversation, and don't realize how much we've eaten.

Have a strategy. Don't go hungry. A couple of pieces of fruit (about 100–150 calories) or a handful of nuts (60 calories) before or on the way to the party will take the edge off your appetite. Compare those with the hors d'oeuvres, one mouthful of which will give you 100 calories. That's especially important if the event begins after your accustomed dinner hour, when you're famished.

Get there late! An untouched buffet table looks so tantalizing. It won't look quite as tempting half an hour later. While you're there, stand as far away from the food table as possible. If you stand alongside it, it's too easy just to reach over and indulge in a few extra bites while you chat. And don't spend much time with someone who's really overweight. They'll probably eat all through the party, and will encourage you to do the same.

A serious reason for eating something before you go is that the affair usually starts with wine or mixed drinks. Alcohol will enter your bloodstream quickly if you haven't eaten for a while. Aside from its effects on your brain, it stimulates the appetite so that you'll eat more of those fatty favorites of every party hostess, and they'll quickly end up as stored body fat.

Have an alcohol strategy. You probably know what your limit is. Most people are measurably impaired after a couple of drinks but almost no one will admit to that. My personal limit is two average sized glasses of wine. From then on it's water, club soda or ginger ale. No one has ever seemed to notice that I've made the switch, perhaps because most of them haven't. When getting a drink that contains hard liquor, ask the bartender for extra ice.

Would Stone-Agers have been chocoholics?

Chocoholics take heart! Your desire for this great gift is quite natural. When our distant relatives, the Incas, the Mayas and the Aztecs, wandered into Central and South America they discovered the tree on which the cocoa bean grows. They treasured it for its aphrodisiac effects, which may have been due more to the pepper and other ingredients that they added to it. Spanish explorers concocted a drink made from powdered cocoa and introduced it to Europe early in the sixteenth century. Three hundred years later an English confectioner invented the chocolate candy that so many of us enjoy almost daily.

Is there a biologic reason for what is nearly an addiction among some people? As scientists uncover more nutritional information about chocolate, that's not at all far-fetched. Among the Cuna Indians of Panama, for example, the dark chocolate that they produce themselves and that they have savored for centuries seems to lower their blood pressure. When they move to urban areas and switch to commercial cocoa preparations, their blood pressure tends to rise. Although researchers attribute the difference to flavonoids that are present in dark chocolate and missing from processed chocolate, I must admit that a move to the city involves other factors that are likely to raise blood pressure, including less physical activity, poor dietary habits and stress.

From a nutritional perspective there is an enormous difference between types of chocolate. Any real benefits apply only to dark chocolate. Chocolate milk and chocolate candy lose most of their nutritional benefits during processing. Most milk chocolate bars contain powdered milk, sugar and saturated fat. White chocolate consists of cocoa butter, sugar, vanilla and milk. Unhealthy trans fats reach high levels in some chocolate-containing baked goods.

More than half the fat in dark chocolate is saturated, but it's of the type called stearic acid that has little or no detrimental effect on cholesterol. Another third is oleic acid, a monounsaturated acid that is also found in olive oil and that has beneficial effects on cholesterol.

Besides fat, dark chocolate contains three groups of substances that could benefit our health: minerals, flavonoids and biogenic amines.

Dark chocolate contains fairly high levels of magnesium. A single serving — about 1½ ounces — provides 15 percent of the recommended daily intake of magnesium, a deficiency of which is associated with high blood pressure, abnormal heart rhythm and stroke. Chocolate also contains other beneficial minerals such as calcium, copper and potassium.

The cocoa bean is, of course, a vegetable, and it contains flavonoids similar to those that occur in apples, onions and wine.

Biogenic amines include caffeine-like substances that stimulate our metabolism. Other members of this group include fatty acids that are related to chemicals in marijuana and which affect mood. These calming amines, as well as magnesium, might explain why chocolate relieves the cravings of women who suffer from pre-menstrual syndrome (PMS).

The fast food follies

Fast food is a boon or a bane, a convenience or a curse, depending on how you make use of it. We spend one-seventh of our food budget at McDonald's and similar places. Nowhere is the mega-sizing of portions as grossly apparent as it is here. In the late 1950s the average-sized hamburger patty weighed barely 2 ounces; now it weighs 6, and double-patties are on every fast food outlet menu. A serving of soda was 8 ounces back then. Now even the "small" sizes are larger than that, the 32-ounce size is common, and 64-ounce containers are so large that they double as advertising signs.

Consumption of soda and fruit drinks has almost doubled in the past generation and milk intake has declined, especially among teenagers. Fast food outlets contribute heavily to this new pattern. There are two reasons why liquid nourishment is adding to dietary imbalance. First, liquids are less satiating than solids, even when the calorie content is identical. Those who drink a calorie-containing beverage during a meal don't compensate by eating less; they simply add the liquid calories. Second, most customers don't recognize the differences between home-sized and restaurant-sized drinks. When asked how many calories are contained in a drink, the usual answer is "about a hundred calories." The responses are the same whether the volume of the serving is 9 ounces or 17 ounces. Form the habit of always asking for the smallest size of any drink, and a glass of water.

Fast food is almost synonymous with fat food. A single meal (hamburger or deep fried chicken or fish, French fries and a milkshake) easily provides a couple of days' worth of the recommended amounts of total fat and saturated fat. Most fast food outlets offer a leafy green salad, but it's rarely possible to get two or three choices of vegetables. Burger sauces are heavy on mayonnaise, which is almost 100 percent fat. Ask to leave them off, and use ketchup instead.

More fast food chains are adding healthier choices to their menus. The difference between these "lite" or "heart healthy" meals and regular items can be 800 calories or more. Just skipping the super-size fries could eliminate 540 calories.

When you travel

Sam and Sal never suffered from jet lag — or airline food. No matter what mode of transportation you choose when you take a trip, unless you plan very carefully you'll skip some meals, snack a lot and settle for foods you'd pass by in other circumstances. A little forethought will help you to avoid hunger, inconvenience, fatigue, and perhaps, even jet lag.

Eat a good breakfast on your day of travel. It may be the only satisfying meal you'll have that day. Eat one or two pieces of fruit during breakfast and take a couple more with you in your carry-on. If your first meal of the day usually includes, or consists of, a couple of cups of coffee, have only one. Caffeine is a diuretic, which means that it will cause you to lose more water than is contained in that cup of coffee. Don't drink coffee on the plane, for the same reason. Tea has a similar but milder effect, so you might want to drink only herb teas on travel days. Drink lots of water during the flight. Even though you'll be in a pressurized cabin, it's set at 10,000 feet, not sea level, and that altitude has a dehydrating effect. Dryness is why mountain powder snow is so light and fluffy. Don't let your body get that way.

Quality food bars are better than the spur-of-the-moment snacks you (over)pay for in the terminal. They have balanced nutrients, and those with extra protein will keep you more alert. Candy bars and cookies will do just the opposite because they cause a spike in blood sugar and a subsequent letdown. Choose your granola bars carefully. Some are very high in fat calories and sugar.

The major airlines seem to be avoiding serving meals at all whenever they can. If you're fortunate (?) enough to be on a meal flight, order a special meal when you make your reservation. You have a choice of vegetarian, seafood (usually the best choice), kosher, fruit plate and perhaps several others such as gluten-free, low cholesterol, etc.

When you travel a long distance by car it's easy to make poor choices if you don't know the territory. Fast food restaurants are tempting not only because they're familiar, but because a quick meal won't mess up your timetable as much as a leisurely meal at a more elegant eating emporium. I suggest that a traditional menu with more selections will make the trip more pleasant, and not just because of the atmosphere. High-fat, high-sugar fast food fare, accompanied by supersized soft drinks that don't satisfy your appetite, will leave you with a low blood sugar a couple of hours down the highway. Pick a restaurant in which you are likely to find whole grains, fresh fruit, and real vegetables. These foods will give you a more even, nonspiking blood glucose, and no letdown.

Get in the habit of keeping some fresh fruit, nuts and protein bars in a small cooler, even during relatively short trips.

In summary, whether you eat at home or away, you don't have to make extraordinary sacrifices in order to enjoy variety, balance and flavor. In Chapter Seven you'll find how you can also guarantee better than average nutrition.

Seven

Supplements: sense and nonsense

"If you eat a normal diet you don't need to take vitamins." That statement is true, but useless. It is what most physicians, including me, believed until the early 1980s. Some doctors still hold that opinion even though a "normal" diet for humans is no longer available except for the few hunter-gatherer groups that civilization has not yet enlightened. In the past decade there has been a sea-change in physicians' attitudes. Most medical practitioners take a multivitamin as well as antioxidants, but they tend not to spend much time discussing nutrition during patient visits.

Don't judge medical practitioners harshly for their apparent disinterest in nutrition. Most of them feel that they are poorly trained in this area. Medical curricula are so crowded that fewer than 25 percent of medical schools require students to take a course in nutrition, and another 25 percent don't even provide one. Busy practitioners find it difficult to find the time to take a proactive position regarding nutrition. Keeping up with new drugs, new procedures and new regulations cuts deeply into their study routine, and the demands of HMOs limit the time available for nutrition counseling.

This attitude is changing. Physicians now recognize that suboptimal intake of vitamins is common, and is a risk factor for several chronic diseases. During the past two decades it has become clear that simple measurements of vitamin levels in blood are not reliable. Studies that correlate vitamin intake and disease show that cardiovascular disease and cancer of the colon and breast, as well as malformations of the brain and spinal cord in infants, are related to inadequate intake of these nutrients. In its professional journal, the American Medical Association recommends that all persons take a multivitamin/multimineral preparation every day.

For more than a million years, Homo sapiens' body chemistry has been evolving to match his environment. After the Agricultural Revolution, his food choices dropped from hundreds to a few dozen. The switch to farming left us with foods of lesser quality. Sam and Sal's fruits, nuts, roots and vegetables thrived among hundreds of other plant species that contributed to their content of minerals and micronutrients. The soil that nourished them never became exhausted; in a sense, it was always fallow. Irrigation didn't saturate it with salt; Sam didn't taint it with toxins.

Stone-Agers ate a diet richer in vitamins, minerals and antioxidants than we do. They had no nutrient-null foods such as sugar and alcohol, which comprise almost one-third of the average American diet. For them, every mouthful of food contained minerals and micronutrients. How different from today.

What vitamins are — and are not

Vitamins are natural substances that help with the countless chemical processes within our bodies, including building, maintaining and repairing cells. They don't provide energy. That comes from the carbohydrate, protein and fat (macronutrients) that form the bulk of our diet. In addition to being a source of energy, protein is necessary for structural growth and repair. Vitamins are micronutrients; we need them only in small but critical amounts. A Dutch physician, Christiaan Eijkman, noted in 1890 that wealthy Indonesians developed beriberi, but poorer ones did not. The rich could afford polished rice from which the hulls had been removed. Those homely husks contained important nutrients. A few years later a Polish chemist, Casimir Funk, identified the first of the B vitamins. Within a couple of decades scientists had identified almost all the vitamins we know today. During the past 50 years researchers have discovered many other microcomponents of foods, some of which may be as important as vitamins in preventing or postponing degenerative diseases, slowing the aging process, protecting pregnancy and preventing birth defects. Their number is enormous, certainly in the thousands. This group of substances is so complex that we may never identify them all, but their interaction is vital to all life processes.

It's important to understand that vitamins are components of natural foods. They are not medicines, although physicians sometimes prescribe them in relatively high doses to treat conditions such as high blood pressure. If taken in great excess they sometimes have significant side effects.

People frequently ask me if natural vitamins are really better than synthetic versions. To address the issue of natural versus synthetic, consider how Sam and Sal obtained their vitamins. These micronutrients exist in the company of hundreds of cofactors that are also present in fruits, vegetables, dairy products and meat, and do not act alone. For instance, researchers have found that there are about 8 milligrams of vitamin C in an apple, but the total amount of antioxidant activity in that fruit is equivalent to about 1,500 milligrams of vitamin C. Many of the flavonoids, flavones, phenols and carotenes function in concert with vitamins, although scientists have not yet determined precisely how. We know that synthetic forms of vitamin E do not always work like the natural version. The hundreds of other micronutrients that were formed along with vitamins in the growing plant are not present when manufacturers make vitamins from simpler chemicals in the laboratory. For some synthetic vitamins that may not matter much, because they will encounter within the body the co-factors they require. In some cases the insufficiency of trace minerals, carotenes, flavonoids, etc., might lead to poorer performance of the vitamin in question. The answer then is a qualified "Yes, provided that their natural cofactors accompany them." My first choice is always the natural vitamin-containing food. My second choice is a vitamin that has been extracted from natural sources and that is accompanied by at least some of its co-factors.

Antioxidants

Free radicals are unstable chemicals that result from the natural processes in our own bodies as we use oxygen and from environmental pollution, atmospheric radiation, sunlight and cigarette smoke. They contribute to heart disease, cancer, cataracts and aging, and are linked to numerous other illnesses. Antioxidants counteract the damaging effects of free radicals. Some vitamins, such as vitamin C and E, have antioxidant properties, but not all do. Many antioxidants, such as Coenzyme Q-10, are not vitamins.

Tomatoes contain lycopene, apples contain quercetin, and green leafy vegetables contain many other antioxidants. Some foods that are among the highest in their antioxidant capacity include prunes, raisins, blueberries, kale and spinach, but these are not common in the average American diet. Each contains dozens, if not hundreds, of antioxidants in addition to those I have named.

Sam and Sal ate an abundance of fruits and vegetables, the best source of antioxidants. It was a diet to which their body chemistry was perfectly adapted by evolution. Modern man not only takes in fewer natural antioxidants, but his sources are not as rich in these chemicals, and his environment has changed drastically in the past few centuries.

Beyond beriberi: what's a vitamin deficiency?

Since I started my medical career more than 45 years ago I have never seen a patient with beriberi, scurvy or pellagra. These three vitamin deficiency diseases take up 43 pages in my oldest medical textbook and less than a single page in the newest. The classic vitamin deficiencies have sunk below medicine's horizon, except for occasional alcoholics and persons with unusual lifestyles.

Today's vitamin-related diseases are better described as inadequacies, not deficiencies. An automobile engine that is deficient in fuel simply stops running. When we fill our car's gas tank with gasoline that is inadequate (i.e., has a lower octane than that which the manufacturer recommends), the motor may "ping," get poorer mileage and require more frequent maintenance. This is similar to what we do to our bodies when we substitute fast food, vitamin-free soft drinks and condensed calories for fresh fruit, lightly or uncooked vegetables and nutritious nuts like the ones that Sam and Sal enjoyed.

There are many reasons why we should supplement our diet with vitamins, minerals and antioxidants. The conditions that I listed above should be enough for most people. I encourage you to take a daily multivitamin-multimineral supplement in moderate amounts. Quality multivitamin preparations contain several antioxidants, such as lutein, quercetin, lipoic acid, lycopene and pycnogenol, among others.

I won't catalog all the known vitamins, describe their function or recommend dosages in these pages. Anyone interested in such details can consult the books I have listed in Appendix 4.

Who needs supplements?

In 1994 the United States Department of Agriculture published a report showing that the average American woman took in less than the recommended daily intake for calcium, magnesium, zinc and iron, as well as vitramin B6 and vitamin E. Among a group of more than 21,500 persons, not a single one consumed 100 percent of the RDA for 10 important nutrients. These included vitamins A, B1, B2, B6, B12, and C, as well as calcium, magnesium, iron and protein.When a study showed that folic acid deficiency increased the risk of fetal brain and spinal cord defects, some doubted it. Subsequent studies clearly confirmed the first, and in 1998 the federal government ordered that folic acid must be included in all cereal and grain products sold in the United States. The reason? The discovery that less than 10 percent of women of childbearing age take the recommended amount, 400 micrograms daily, of folic acid. Inadequate folic acid during pregnancy may also be related to defects of the limbs, urinary tract, lip and palate.

> The average American diet contains approximately half the recommended amount of folic acid in spite of its addition to grains and cereal products.

The need for folic acid does not end at birth. Physicians identified it as a critical factor for healthy blood cells more than 50 years ago. More recently it has become evident that folic acid has a role in disorders of the adult brain, including depression in the elderly. A low intake of folic acid increases the risk of cardiovascular disease, as well as cancer of the colon and breast.

Aging and vitamin needs

Respected academic physicians make it clear that vitamin deficiencies are common, especially among the elderly. Older people tend to eat less, partly because they begin to lose their sense of taste and smell, but taking in fewer calories doesn't reduce their need for vitamins and minerals. Those who have lost some of their natural teeth have lower intakes of several nutrients. If they live alone they find cooking a chore. When they aren't feeling well because of so-called age-related illnesses, they won't take the time to prepare a nutritious meal. They have more stress because of insecurity and loneliness and financial problems. As they age they don't absorb vitamins as well, especially vitamin B12. The elderly are more likely to be taking prescription drugs, some of which interfere with absorption of vitamins.

Diseases of the heart and blood vessels have multiple causes. Homocysteine is an amino acid, albeit a harmful one, which increases in the elderly. As homocysteine levels rise, so does the risk of coronary heart disease.

The immune system has several components that are dispersed throughout the body. Taken together, they form a large organ and require a considerable share of the energy and the micronutrients we take in every day. Immune function declines as individuals age. One possible cause is the accumulation of environmental toxins over decades. The lower antioxidant level among older persons, coupled with an excess of omega-6 fatty acids (see below) might further compromise their immune systems. Zinc deficiency compromises the immune system even further, and in persons over the age of 60, up to 90 percent are deficient in this important nutrient.

Our cellular immune system is that which helps us to overcome several kinds of infectious diseases, such as fungus infections and tuberculosis. When healthy-appearing older persons take a multivitamin supplement the response of their cellular immune system improves. The addition of vitamin E to the diet also improves cellular immune responses, and enhances the body's production of antibodies to the hepatitis B vaccine.

> Do cataracts develop naturally as a result of aging? Perhaps not. A diet that includes multivitamins, including folate, vitamin A and the B group, especially B12, is associated with a lower incidence of cataracts.

Young adults and vitamin needs

Women who are taking birth control pills or who are pregnant have increased vitamin needs. So do men and women who exercise, as well as those who drink any amount of alcohol. It's hard to eat properly during travel, whether by plane or by car. Individuals on a diet need a full complement of vitamins and minerals; they require even more antioxidants because of the stress that accompanies fasting.

Smokers expose themselves to a large number of toxic chemicals that cause short-term and long-term damage to cells, not just within the lungs but also throughout the body. Tobacco smoke contains numerous oxidants, and the blood of smokers is low in antioxidants. Smokers also tend to have a lower intake of fruits and vegetables that might provide them with antioxidants. Taking supplements, especially those that contain vitamin C, can restore their antioxidant levels.

Children and vitamin needs

The ardor of those who promote long-term breast-feeding of infants is justified, but it does not mean that breastmilk has all the vitamins a child requires. That depends on the adequacy of the mother's diet. If she falls in the large category of American adults whose vitamin intake is below recommended levels, her milk will reflect that. As an example, vitamin D-deficient rickets, a disease that most pediatricians in this country have never seen, is returning. The rarity of rickets in the recent past is a major problem; most physicians will not recognize its early signs. As the rate of breast-feeding increases, the fact that many pediatricians do not recommend vitamin supplementation for nursing infants means that we will see more cases of this disease in the coming years. All breastfed infants should receive a daily multivitamin preparation.

French fries comprise about one-quarter of the vegetables in children's diets. Only 1 in 5 children eats 5 or more servings of fruits and vegetables per day. In 1970, children drank twice as much milk as soda; by 2000 that ratio was reversed. Every parent knows that it's almost impossible to get a three-year-old to eat anything green or yellow unless it's candy or Jell-O. (Not that adults are much better. According to the USDA in their 1994 survey, only 1 in 7 adults had eaten deep yellow vegetables recently and only about 1 in 9 had eaten dark green vegetables.) Mothers who make a nutritious sandwich for their children sometimes find out that the youngster traded it at school for a few cookies or a candy bar.

> *Nature is not on mother's side. The 5 most nutritious vegetables are broccoli, spinach, Brussels sprouts, lima beans and peas. They provide generous amounts of vitamins A and C, niacin, thiamine and riboflavin, as well as potassium, calcium and iron. And most kids hate them.*

Do vitamin supplements improve a child's intelligence? The answer is that they do in a subset of children whose diet is inadequate, but the improvement is not dramatic. Most studies were carried out over a period of just a few weeks.

Nutritional trends among children are going in the wrong direction. They are eating fewer fruits and vegetables than in decades past, they are becoming more obese, and their milk intake is declining. We can provide them with supplements now, but reforming their dietary habits will be a long-term challenge.

A stacked deck

The most ardent supporters of supplementation urge us to get our vitamins, minerals and antioxidants from natural foods, and I agree with them. Unfortunately, we can no longer duplicate the nutrient content of the foods that Sam and Sal ate. Further, contemporary Homo sapiens has micronutrient requirements that didn't exist when man's metabolism was evolving. High stress levels and environmental toxins are just two examples. First, let's consider how our food supply has changed.

Soil depletion (Chapter One) began when the first farmer sowed his second crop in the same location as the previous year. It probably took many generations before primitive agriculturalists figured out that nutrients must be returned to the soil, and that one way to do this was to allow fields to remain fallow, or uncultivated, for a time. Irrigation enlarged the area of arable land, but it also produced a gradual buildup of salt that eventually reduced crop yields below those that could sustain the population.

Modern farmers in the Imperial Valley of Southern California have not yet found the answer to this 10,000-year-old problem. They plant salt-resistant crops and install expensive drainage systems, but these are only temporary solutions.

Commercial growers cannot afford to allow the biblical one-seventh of their land to remain unused, so they pour tons of synthetic fertilizer onto every arable acre. They can maintain the quantity of their yields this way, but not the quality that nature provides. Under natural conditions, wild flora and fauna exist in a mutually helpful state. When plants wither and decay they provide nutrients for the ones that grow up in their place. Animals and insects contribute waste matter during life and bodily compost after death. From the beginning of agriculture, farmers unknowingly but systematically undid what nature took thousands of years to accomplish. Consider what happened in the lands around the Mediterranean Sea. As the population grew it needed wood for building and fuel, as well as charcoal for the production of metal implements. The forests of Greece and other lands provided it. When the trees were gone the scant rainfall couldn't support regrowth. At about the same time, hunters realized that it was easier to capture and corral wild goats than to hunt them. Goats ate the vegetation that held the topsoil in place. Wind and water removed the loosened soil and within a few hundred years most of the forests and many plants were gone. The mischief that man set in motion around the Mediterranean and in the Middle East he has duplicated around the globe. In his televised documentary, *Earth on Edge* (June 19, 2001), journalist Bill Moyers noted that every acre of farmland in Kansas loses 7 tons of topsoil each year. Soil depletion is a fact of agricultural life, and no manufactured nutrients can match nature's.

Zinc deficiency is a classical example of the effect of soil depletion. Around the shores of the Mediterranean Sea, where farmers have grown wheat for more than 4,000 years, dwarfism is common in males. Adding zinc to the diet eliminates this aberrant growth pattern.

When I was in grade school we lived near an abandoned orchard. I'd spend a few hours at the end of the summer sitting beneath or climbing among the branches of the apple trees, enjoying my private harvest. Only the worms had apples fresher than mine. Whenever I bite into a mealy apple now I wonder when it was picked, how long it has been in a warehouse, and what has been done to it to keep it from rotting. Flavor fades when fruits are stored; so does their nutritional value. Vitamin C levels drop within hours.

Sam and Sal had no means of preserving vegetables, so what they ate was usually fresh. Our produce is almost always a day or two old. Food producers who can harvest and process their product rapidly may provide us with better nutrition than the local farmer whose vegetables arrive at the market a day or two after harvest.

Frozen vegetables usually retain more vitamins than those that are canned if they are harvested at their peak of freshness and processed quickly. Storing uncooked vegetables for a prolonged period may cause them to lose more vitamins than some processed foods.

Early humans ate most of their foods raw, for they had little choice. They learned how to control fire more than 700,000 years ago but their use of cooking utensils was far in the future. We eat most of our vegetables, and almost all our meat, after we have cooked it. Heating reduces the vitamin content of most foods and boiling water accelerates the loss. For instance, when we boil a potato we lower the vitamin C level by about half and the folate by about 25 percent. Canning also diminishes the vitamin content of food. Samples of canned peas show losses of vitamin C as high as 64 percent.

Some special nutrients in perspective

There is a time lag in the dissemination of medical information. New discoveries, unless commercial interests drive them, tiptoe slowly into clinical practice. When fresh findings run up against entrenched dogma, especially when their benefits are unspectacular and lack financial incentive, they must creep into the tent of the medical establishment. The nutrients I discuss below have a mixed history but they share one common characteristic: few Americans obtain adequate amounts in their diet, because even fewer physicians recommend their use. Practitioners recognized decades ago that calcium and vitamin D had critical roles in bone health. Nevertheless, more than half of those persons who need them fail to take the recommended daily intake. Studies on vitamin E are inconsistent. Vitamin C's champion was an iconoclastic nonagenarian, a Nobel laureate whose personality and politics shrouded his scientific accomplishments. Omega-3 fatty acids are Johnnies-come-lately onto the medical scene. All these nutrients deserve some special attention.

The vitamin E shortfall

The new RDI (Recommended Dietary Intake) of vitamin E is 22 units daily, but most Americans take much less. Researchers in the field take several times that much themselves, about 400 units per day. Some recommend 800. In two studies involving more than

120,000 people, researchers found that large doses of vitamin E are associated with a significantly decreased risk of coronary artery disease. Yet, academic physicians continue to oppose the use of supplements, and still prefer the use of cholesterol-lowering agents in spite of the fact that pharmaceutical companies have recalled several of these because of serious, sometimes fatal, side effects. In doses below 800 units per day vitamin E has no significant toxicity. A dosage of 400 units a day is safe, but most multivitamin combinations do not contain that much. In order to get 400 units of vitamin E from dietary sources it would be necessary to eat several hundred calories of fat-containing foods.

You could get 400 units of natural vitamin E by eating all of the following vitamin E-rich foods every day:

1.3 bowls of Total brand cereal
6 tablespoons of safflower oil
66 tablespoons of mayonnaise
1 pound of dried almonds
36 cups of kale

You'd also be getting about 10,700 calories!

How could Sam and Sal have gotten that much vitamin E? They probably didn't, nor did they have to. Modern circumstances have determined these recommendations in order to protect us against conditions that didn't exist back then. Fifty thousand years ago there was no tobacco smoke or automobile exhaust, no factory emissions or industrial contamination of drinking water. The ozone layer was intact and the stress our ancestors encountered was occasional, not constant.

Sam and Sal had only about a 1 in 10 chance of living past the age of 60, but this is the fastest-growing age group among Western nations. Damaged proteins accumulate as we get older, we produce fewer antioxidants, and we become more vulnerable to free-radical damage. There is much dispute regarding the effectiveness of vitamin E taken as a supplement, perhaps because of the wide variation in the type, source and amount of the product.

Vitamin E in a capsule is not the same as vitamin E in natural foods. There are 8 different forms of this antioxidant in nature. The best supplements include mixed tocopherols, or d-alpha tocopherol. The synthetic version, dl-alpha tocopherol, has about one-half the activity of natural forms.

Vitamin C, the antioxidant workhorse

Vitamin C appears to work together with vitamin E, especially in protecting us against cancer and diseases of the heart and blood vessels. It is also one of the most controversial vitamins, and arguments continue to rage regarding the optimum dosage, or even whether supplements are necessary at all. Sam and Sal probably took about 160 milligrams of vitamin C per day, almost 3 times the current Recommended Daily Intake (RDI). Many authorities recommend 500 to 1,000 milligrams (mg.) per day. This is a safe dosage but it may cause stomach discomfort in some persons.

Smokers tend to have lower vitamin C levels than nonsmokers. Tobacco smoke has a direct toxic effect on the inner lining of blood vessels, probably because it has high concentrations of free radicals and other damaging substances. Vitamin C has a direct effect on restoring circulation in small blood vessels of the heart that have been damaged by tobacco smoke.

The last generation has seen a marked increase in the incidence of asthma in children as well as adults. Like so many chronic diseases, asthma has a variety of causes. Some studies show that a diet that is low in vitamin C is one of the risk factors for this disease, and in adult-onset asthma, supplementation with antioxidants is associated with a lessening of symptoms.

Mediterranean people have a relatively high intake of vitamin C. They also have a high prevalence of smoking, but their incidence of coronary artery disease is lower than that of persons who live in northern Europe.

Vitamin D — where it fits in the big picture

In order to understand vitamin D we need to have a better understanding of what really causes osteoporosis. There's more to preventing this crippling condition than taking calcium. As I noted in Chapter Four, weight-bearing exercise is a key factor. It is largely for that reason that persons living in poor countries, with the lowest intake of calcium, also have the lowest incidence of hip fractures.

Consider your skeleton as a framework of fibers to which you add calcium. Protein is a key factor because it makes up those fibers, as well as the blood vessels that nourish the entire structure. Contrary to older studies, new ones show that a moderately high intake of protein yields greater bone density. Although protein can lead to a loss of calcium, it does so only when it is highly purified or is eaten in amounts far above normal.

As an example of how complex this disorder is, new studies show that high levels of homocysteine weaken this protein network. A generous intake of fruits and vegetables, a recurring theme in this book, lowers homocysteine levels

Magnesium, which is abundant in fruits or vegetables, is also a vital factor in normal bone development and maintenance. So is boron, which has only recently received much study. About six prunes will provide you with the recommended daily dose of boron, but you'd probably enjoy getting it more from other good sources such as red wine, almonds or raisins. So would I.

Vitamin D helps to maintain bone by increasing our ability to absorb calcium and phosphorus from the food we eat. In addition, it increases the activity of cells called *osteoblasts* that build and reshape our skeleton throughout our entire life. This continuing remodeling process needs other cells that dissolve bone and release calcium into the bloodstream. A deficiency of vitamin D allows these *osteoclasts* to gain the upper hand. That makes the bones become softer, a condition called osteomalacia. Not only does this lead to fractures, it causes muscle pain and weakness that is often misdiagnosed as fibromyalgia.

Osteoporosis is not so simple. In osteoporosis the framework itself, as described above, is deficient because of the lack of several nutrients, not just calcium. In many women it begins in adolescence because of a combination of inactivity and inadequate nutrition. With continued lack of exercise in adult life the very structure of bone becomes thin and fragile, and it breaks easily.

Vitamin D has other important duties to carry out, such as helping to maintain the immune system and inhibit the growth of cancer. It lowers blood pressure and brings blood sugar (glucose) down in patients with diabetes.

The elderly are most likely to get inadequate amounts of vitamin D. This is, of course, the group in which osteoporosis and hip fractures contribute so much to a poor quality of life and premature death. They tend to have poor nutrition habits, spend more time indoors than younger persons, and be more likely to have chronic diseases involving the liver and kidney. They worry more about skin cancer and keep their skin covered when they do venture outdoors. All these factors contribute to the development of low levels of vitamin D, and the older the patient, the greater the risk.

Nature designed us to get vitamin D from the sun, not from our diet, but living in a sunny part of the world is no guarantee that you can avoid vitamin D deficiency. If you live north of a line drawn from Atlanta to Los Angeles you may not get the sun exposure you need, especially during the winter. In the northernmost latitudes of the United States and Canada almost no one gets enough vitamin D from sun exposure for half the year.

For persons over the age of 50, the National Academy of Sciences recommends 400 units per day, and 600 units for those over the age of 70. An eight-ounce glass of milk contains about 100 units of vitamin D, but most of us, especially the elderly, don't get even that much. Repeated surveys of persons over the age of 50 show that more than half fail to make enough or eat enough of this important vitamin all year long.

Foods such as salmon, sardines, eggs and fortified cereals contain some vitamin D, but it's simply impossible to get enough from dietary sources. I highly recommend a supplement of 400 units for all ages, but not to exceed 800 units except under a doctor's supervision. All breastfed babies should also receive vitamin D according to the recommendation of their pediatrician.

Calcium

If you've reached the age of 50 you may already be receiving the monthly publication of the AARP (American Association of Retired Persons) with its regular reminders that you need to take at least 1,000 milligrams of calcium daily in order to avoid osteoporosis. They're a little late. The best time to build up protection from that bone-thinning condition is during adolescence and early adulthood. Sam and Sal took large amounts of calcium, more than 1,500 milligrams daily, from their mostly vegetarian food supply. Our diet contains fewer vegetables, and the grain products we eat in their place contain less calcium. Further, the calcium in grains is not as available for absorption from the intestine as that which is found in vegetables.

This mineral is the one most often lacking in the average diet, especially among persons who eat few dairy products. Those on a weight reduction diet, particularly women, usually don't keep up with their calcium needs when they cut back on their total food intake. Reducing calories doesn't reduce the need for essential minerals. According to the United States Department of Agriculture, 90 percent of adult women and teenage girls and 75 percent of men don't get the recommended daily intake of this essential nutrient. That's no surprise, considering how far we have wandered from the Stone Age diet. Remember that Sam and Sal didn't eat dairy products at all, because there were none. Their calcium came from green plants, which is the same source from which cows get it. Most physicians recommend milk and cheese as sources of calcium, but many adults cannot tolerate lactose, the sugar in milk. A high intake of dairy products, with their high level of fat, is one of the reasons Americans are overweight.

The value of calcium extends far beyond healthy bones. It has a key role in the health of muscle, including the heart muscle. It is probably more important than sodium in controlling blood pressure. Calcium, especially in the form of low-fat dairy products, accelerates fat loss in persons on a low-calorie diet.

Almost everyone needs to take a calcium supplement. That is so not only because the average daily intake in the United States is less than half that which the Recommended Daily Intake calls for, but because so few people exercise, as noted in Chapter Four. The specific form (carbonate or citrate) really doesn't matter. The difference in their rates of absorption is inconsequential. We only absorb about half our calcium intake no matter what form it's in.

Don't be misled by the argument that too much calcium causes kidney stones. That simply is not true. You will not find excessive calcium intake on the list of the causes of kidney stones in any medical text. Among 45,000 men studied at the Harvard School of Public Health, those with the highest calcium intake had the lowest incidence of kidney stones. Restricting calcium intake actually increases the risk of forming kidney stones. Although many types of kidney stones contain calcium, it's due to other factors, not excessive dietary intake. There's a limit to how much calcium we can absorb from the intestines, and any excess intake simply passes through.

Omega-3 fatty acids come of age[1]

Interest in the omega-3 fatty acids began to rise in the 1970s when researchers found that the Inuit natives of Greenland had a very low rate of heart attacks. This was hard to explain because they ate a diet high in fat and low in vegetables. A lower rate of coronary artery disease, and especially less risk of sudden death from a heart attack, was also observed in the Japanese and other population groups. A high intake of fish seems to be the common denominator. Several carefully controlled studies of omega-3 fatty acids, primary components of fish fat, showed dramatic reductions in abnormal heart rhythms and sudden death in persons who ate fish or included fish oil in their diet.

There are more than 6,000 published scientific articles on this large and complex group of fats. Most of them show significant health benefits among persons who have a high, i.e., normal, intake of omega fatty acids in the correct proportion. They are called essential fatty acids, but even that term seems like an understatement. They contribute to the stability and flexibility of almost every cell in our body, and have other properties as well. It's no wonder that the list of problems associated with inadequate intake or imbalance is so long. It includes coronary and cerebral thrombosis (heart attack and stroke), high blood pressure, osteoarthritis, immune-inflammatory diseases such as systemic lupus erythematosus and rheumatoid arthritis, Crohn's disease, asthma, various brain disorders, postpartum depression, premature birth, and cancers of the breast, colon and prostate. These diseases are infrequent or rare in Japanese, who take in about 4 ½ times as much fish

[1] From: O'Keefe JH and Harris WS, "From Inuit to Implementation: Omega-3 Fatty Acids Come of Age," *Mayo Clinic Proceedings* June 2000; 75:607–614.

fat as Americans, and among native Greenlanders, whose intake of protective omega-3s is 15 times higher than ours.

Omega-3 and omega-6 fatty acids belong to a large group of polyunsaturated fats, so called because they have room for more hydrogen atoms, which would make them saturated, like animal fat. The body forms prostaglandins, chemicals that influence inflammation and numerous other processes, from both types of omega fatty acids. In general, prostaglandins from omega-3s lead to reduced inflammation; the ones made from omega-6s contribute to inflammation. We need about equal amounts of omega-3s and omega-6s; imbalance leads to disease. Sam and Sal had a plentiful supply of each, but their ratio of omega-6s to omega-3s was about 1:1. That's because they didn't have vegetable oils, which are a major (and excessive) source of omega-6s for us. Their omega-3s came from fish, nuts, leafy greens and wild game. Most of the farm-raised meat and fish in our markets comes from animals that have no access to natural foods, and the grain that is used to feed them has little omega-3 fatty acid. Thus, not only do we get too little omega-3s because we don't eat the kind of food our ancestors did, we get an excess of omega-6s because we eat foods they never dreamed of. Instead of a 1:1 ratio, ours is about 15:1 in favor of omega-6s.

Farm-raised fish and eggs could give us more omega-3s if breeders provided the proper ingredients in feed. The same is true of poultry, pork and beef. These changes will not occur until there is an informed and demanding public.

During the past two decades there has been a massive surge in interest among health authorities and research scientists regarding these polyunsaturated fatty acids, their precursors, their derivatives, and the diseases and conditions with which they are associated. In spite of this, retail medicine has not yet gotten the message. The foremost textbook of medicine contains only 84 words on omega-3 fatty acids among its 2,629 pages. Breastmilk contains 30 times as much omega-3 fatty acid as cow's milk and has significant beneficial effects on eye and brain development in children. Yet, the leading textbook of pediatrics does not list them in the index and only discusses fatty acids in a section on inherited defects.

The Lacustrine[2] leap

After making little intellectual and developmental progress for about 2 million years, early Homo sapiens began, in evolutionary terms, a burst of brain growth and sophistication in tool making. These changes probably began more than 400,000 years ago and accelerated about 100,000 years ago. The period coincides with his greater presence near the lakes and rivers of East Africa, where skeletons and tools provide a record of these advances. In his dwelling sites and middens (scientific vernacular for trash heaps) anthropologists have found huge amounts of shells and fish bones. They have identified fish scales in the coprolites (fossilized feces) of that era.

Marine foods have an abundance of DHA, an omega-3 fatty acid of critical importance to brain development, whereas plant foods do not. This may explain why the large land animals of Africa, with their great body mass, have relatively small brains. One of the largest, the rhinoceros, has a brain that makes up only 0.1 percent of its weight. For a plant-eater closer to man's lineage, the gorilla, it is only 0.25 percent. A human brain represents 2 percent of body mass.

A diet rich in omega-3 fatty acids may have allowed the brain of Homo sapiens to grow in size and complexity. Some scientists have noted that other species of Homo, such as Homo ergaster and Homo rudolfensis, who did not partake of the marine harvest, became evolutionary dead-ends because they were unable to compete with sapiens.

The lacustrine theory may explain why human civilizations have clustered near shorelines for thousands of years. No lasting

2
  From *lacus*, the Latin word for lake. The anthropological term includes the marine environment.

Fat facts

DHA is docosahexaenoic acid. EPA is eicosapentaenoic acid. Both are omega-3s. They are formed from linolenic acid, one of the essential fatty acids, which means that we cannot make it in our bodies, but must have it in our diet. The other essential fatty acid is linoleic, an omega-6 that forms arachidonic acid, another omega-6. (If you wonder why scientists gave them such similar and confusing names, linolenic and linoleic, I've puzzled over that since medical school.)

---

cultures have survived where fish and shellfish are not available. The omega-3 fatty acids don't get all the credit. Iodine is a critical nutrient for brain development. In undeveloped mountainous areas mental deficiency is common. Indeed, the World Health Organization identifies iodine deficiency as the leading cause of mental retardation. Some 1.6 billion people remain at risk, most of them living inland, or on waterways and flood plains that have been leached by rain.

I noted earlier that we can no longer obtain many of the micro-nutrients our bodies require without supplementing our diet. Omega-3 fatty acids are an exception. Only 3 or 4 servings of cold-water fish per week will provide us with the recommended dose of 650 to 1,000 milligrams per day (average) of the two most important omega-3 fatty acids, EPA and DHA, or their precursors. The higher dose is recommended for those at greater than average risk of heart attack or stroke. The best sources are salmon, sardines, herring, mackerel, albacore and anchovy. Shellfish, sole, tuna and swordfish contain less than the others, but are still worthwhile components of our diet. Vegetable sources are less generous in their yield, and include soybeans and soybean oil, flaxseeds and flaxseed oil, nuts (especially walnuts), and leafy green vegetables. There is no need to hunt for sources of omega-6 fatty acids; they are already overabundant in our diet.

> You can find which companies have submitted their products for quality testing at www.consumerlab.com. Be wary of companies that have not done so.

The wide selection of fish that we have in our markets and the innumerable recipes available should make it your first choice as a source of omega-3 fatty acids. Those who dislike fish have a selection of flaxseed or fish oil supplements. Cod liver oil is a last resort. There is just no way to make cod liver oil taste good, and it contains too much vitamin A to be taken in large quantities.

Pregnant women, for whom omega-3 fatty acids are especially important, may have to search beyond fish for their supply. The Environmental Protection agency and some international organizations caution that pregnant women should limit their fish intake. There are rising levels of toxins like methyl mercury and PCBs (polychlorinated biphenyls) in the larger species of fish (www.epa.gov/ost/fishadvice). Fish oil supplements could theoretically be contaminated with these toxins. You should only purchase them from reliable companies that

> Omega-3 fatty acids and their precursors are as vital in maintaining bone mass in elderly persons as calcium and exercise.

maintain high quality control standards. Freshwater fish may also contain PCBs. Women should avoid uncooked shellfish during pregnancy and lactation because of a high risk of contamination with hepatitis virus and other microorganisms. Supplements derived from flaxseed, algae and salmon may be the best choice for pregnant and lactating women.

Quality pays; pay for quality

Vitamin supplements are usually produced under food quality standards, which require less stringent criteria for potency and purity. Few companies operate under pharmaceutical standards, which are more demanding and more expensive. When independent laboratories test vitamin products it is not unusual to find that a given preparation contains much less of the target ingredient than that which is listed on the label. In a few cases it may contain none at all.

Cheaper products may not be stable. Some don't dissolve within the stomach and intestines, so their contents can't be absorbed.

The matter of herbal supplements is beyond the scope of this book. Without doubt, Sam and Sal had a huge natural pharmacy that included herbs. During the middle of the twentieth century, mainstream medicine shunned "natural" medicines, somehow ignoring the fact that until then, natural plant sources provided most of the drugs doctors were using. Early modern antibiotics, anti-inflammatory and anticancer agents came from plant substances. It's also true that irresponsible, unethical and overzealous practitioners have misused herbal treatments. New scientific methods will certainly lead to the rediscovery of some of the genuinely useful medicines of the Stone Age healer, just as nutritionists are uncovering the benefits of the Stone Age diet.

To summarize, a high intake of fruits and vegetables is the starting point to obtain adequate micronutrients. I hope that I have adequately presented sufficient information to help you to make a decision about your need for vitamin and mineral supplementation. In order to ensure that you have adequate micronutrients every day of your life, I suggest a quality multivitamin, one that gives at least the Recommended Daily Intake (RDI) for vitamins A, C, D and E, folic acid and the B-complex group. Those who are unwilling or unable to eat dairy products should take a calcium supplement. The best regimen for a proper balance of fatty acids is a diet rich in vegetables and cold-water fish, or the equivalent in supplements. Vitamins C (1,000 milligrams) and E (400 units) are essential antioxidants that are harmless in the doses I recommend.

Trace minerals such as copper, zinc and cobalt, antioxidants such as quercetin and lutein, and other micronutrients have well-established roles in human nutrition. If you will follow the guidelines above you will have an adequate supply of them.

Eight

In the house of tomorrow:
start with the children

And a woman, who held a babe against
her bosom said, Speak to us of Children.
And he said:
Your children are not your children.
They are the sons and daughters of Life's longing for itself.
They come through you but not from you,
And though they are with you yet they belong not to you.

You may give them your love but not your thoughts,
For they have their own thoughts.
You may house their bodies but not their souls,
For their souls dwell in the house of
tomorrow, which you cannot visit, not even in your dreams.
You may strive to be like them, but seek
Not to make them like you.
For life goes not backward nor tarries with yesterday.

From *The Prophet*, by Kahlil Gibran,
Alfred A. Knopf, publ., New York

Homo sapiens survived and thrived because he adapted so well to his environment, which until barely 100,000 years ago was limited to temperate zones. This territory, between south-central Africa, the western shores of Europe and the eastern edge of Asia, held varied and abundant vegetation and wild game. Early humans faced daily dangers. Most of Sam and Sal's contemporaries died of infection and injury before they saw 40 season-cycles. For the same reasons, average life expectancy barely budged throughout that slender slice of time from the beginning of the Agricultural Revolution to the mid-1800s. Malnutrition and epidemic disease, the one adding to the misery of the other, limited man's population, progress and lifespan.

Life expectancy has increased — almost doubled — in the last couple of centuries. The plumbers of the world deserve credit for the earlier improvements, physicians for the later ones. If we are to make more progress, it will come through making lifestyle changes. Health authorities know how difficult that is. Our best chance is to start with the children.

Every pediatrician knows that children are not just little adults, but physicians who deal with children are seeing adult-type diabetes in preteens. Pediatric pathologists find changes in the coronary arteries of young people that earlier examiners did not discover until the fourth or fifth decade of life. Obesity is the most common thread that leads to 4 of the major causes of death in the United States: heart disease, cancer, stroke and diabetes. It is a preventable process that begins before the first egg leaves the ovary of the mother-to-be.

Sal and Baby Sally

A healthy pregnancy doesn't begin at the moment of conception; it begins during the mother's childhood years. Sal would have been an obstetrician's dream patient. Her family was part of a band that migrated along the northwestern coast of the Mediterranean Sea, and Sal helped to collect food and carry supplies as soon as she was able. The men of her band were skillful hunters and rarely came home without fresh meat. This and the fruits, nuts and vegetables that made up the remainder of her diet were rich in protein, carbohydrate, calcium, vitamins and essential fatty acids. When the fertilized egg — baby Sally — attached itself to the luxuriant lining of Sal's womb, it was off to a healthy start.

The daily intake of the average American is deficient in several important nutrients and we should not be surprised that pregnant women follow the same pattern. Pregnant adolescents are still growing themselves, so their nutritional deficiencies are magnified. This may be one of the factors that make the risk of pregnancy greater among teenagers. Only 11 percent of pregnant adolescents have an adequate intake of vitamin D and only 6 percent of them meet the daily requirements for iron. Less than a third take in the recommended amounts of vitamin E, calcium and magnesium.

The pregnant and breastfeeding mother's need for calcium increases in order to meet the demands of the child she carries and nourishes. If her intake is not high enough the fetus will draw calcium from the mother's bones. If a woman has not developed a strong skeleton during adolescence through vigorous activity and a sufficient diet, she will lose bone mass during pregnancy and lactation, contributing to the osteoporosis that will threaten her own well-being in the future. Sal and her Stone Age contemporaries had a calcium intake that was approximately double that of modern Americans, and their active lifestyle helped them to develop a large bone mass at an early age. Their calcium intake came from fruits and vegetables, not from grain, so that more of it was absorbed.

After weaning a woman will make up for the calcium lost during pregnancy and lactation, but only if her dietary intake of this mineral is normal.

Virtually all (99 percent) of an American woman's bone mass is attained by the time she reaches the age of 26; 90 percent is present by the age of 17. Where do today's adolescent girls get their calcium? Not from vegetables, as Sal did, since their intake is so low. The only other significant source is dairy products, yet between 1979 and 1994 the proportion of girls who drank milk fell from 72 percent to 57 percent. During that same period their soft drink consumption rose by 65 percent.

> **Soda now, fracture later**
>
> *Soft drinks have displaced milk in the diet of most American children, so that more than half of teenage girls do not get the recommended daily amount of calcium. Inadequate calcium intake early in life could reduce peak adult bone mass by 5 to 10 percent. That may result in a 50 percent greater risk of hip fracture later in life. The risk of future osteoporosis is even greater in women who become pregnant during adolescence.*

Gestational diabetes is one of the more serious complications of pregnancy. It's characterized by high blood sugar and insulin levels during pregnancy and almost always presages frank type 2 diabetes later in life. Among some population groups the incidence of elevated insulin levels has reached 20 percent by the age of 20 years. This means that an ever-expanding pool of young women is at risk of developing gestational diabetes. It carries a greater likelihood of complications, including a higher rate of Caesarean section.

Barely a generation ago pediatricians never encountered type 2 diabetes in a lifetime of practice. It now comprises about half of all diabetes in children, some of whom become pregnant during their adolescent years. Infants of diabetic mothers have a mortality rate more than 5 times that of nondiabetics, and the incidence of congenital defects is 3 times as high.

The obese pregnant woman endures almost as many complications as the one with gestational diabetes, including high blood pressure, a greater incidence of Caesarean section, problems involving anesthesia and surgery, postoperative infection and gestational diabetes. The child she carries also faces greater risks, among which are difficulty in getting breathing started, fluid retention and spinal cord defects. The greater the mother's BMI (Body Mass Index, see Chapter One), the higher is the risk that her infant will not survive. It's highly unlikely that Sal was obese, or even overweight, but more than half of her present-day descendants are.

During the last 2 months of fetal development, baby Sally's brain and eyes required a large amount of DHA and EPA, the critical omega-3 fatty acids I described in Chapter Seven, and arachidonic acid (AA), an omega-6 form. As in the case of calcium, the fetus preferentially draws these nutrients from the stores of the mother. If she has inadequate supplies, the infant's developing nervous system will not attain its genetically programmed potential. The transfer of DHA (docosahexaenoic acid, one of the critical omega-3 fatty acids) from mother to infant is greatest during the last trimester of pregnancy, which is the period of maximal development of the brain and the retina of the eye. What can be even more serious is that omega-3 fatty acids are important in supporting pregnancy, and that a deficiency of these substances may be partly responsible for premature delivery and the accompanying hazards to the newborn infant.

The strong influence of omega-3 fatty acids on the outcome of pregnancy has stimulated a surge in research, with significant new findings. An increased consumption of these nutrients may be linked to a lower incidence of cerebral palsy, and to a lower risk of cardiovascular disease in adult life.

As physicians have come to recognize the effects of inadequate vitamin intake, the role of micronutrients in pregnancy has come under new study. For example, a lack of vitamin B12 may be associated with the repeated inability to maintain a pregnancy for a full 9 months. Sometimes prematurity is the result of early rupture of the membranes that surround the fetus and shield it from bacteria residing within the lower portion of the birth canal. In addition to the recognized hazards of premature birth, serious, sometimes fatal infection may follow a leak in this protective barrier. Vitamins C and E, acting here as antioxidants, may keep the fetal membranes from the damaging effects of free radicals that accumulate during infection and inflammation.

A high intake of fruits and vegetables may have protected Sal from preeclampsia, a life-threatening complication of pregnancy that may progress to very high blood pressure, seizures and premature labor. Pregnant women with a diet low in vitamin C and other antioxidants have a more than threefold risk of preeclampsia.

The Stone Age diet, which contained no nutrient-null (empty) calories, was so varied that it was not likely to be deficient even in the face of the increased demands of pregnancy. The food intake of Americans is often lacking in important dietary factors, and practitioners who care for pregnant women regularly prescribe a daily multivitamin/multimineral preparation in case there are deficiencies. Not all women receive good prenatal care, nor do they take in even the minimum recommended amount of most vitamins. Investigators at the Centers for Disease Control and Prevention have confirmed previous studies that link severe cardiac defects with inadequate vitamin intake during the periconceptional period. That is the period starting three months before conception through the third month of pregnancy. The particular heart problems observed were *conotruncal* defects. These involve the large blood vessels that leave the heart before they branch off to supply the lungs and the rest of the body. In that study, more than 2,100 infants were born to mothers taking supplemental vitamins. There were only 10 congenital heart defects among those babies, and none were of the conotruncal type. Infants born to mothers not taking multivitamins had almost twice as many heart defects and 2 were of the conotruncal type.

Obesity is a form of malnutrition, and overweight women are more likely to be deficient in vitamins and minerals. The physicians who confirmed the association between inadequate multivitamin intake and heart defects found that overweight women also had an increased risk of delivering a child with a major heart defect. Furthermore, in spite of taking daily supplements, the infants of these women still had a higher percentage of congenital heart abnormalities.

Primitive man began to use fire about one million years ago, although full control probably didn't occur until he developed more sophisticated tools a half-million years later. Shelters with indoor hearths must have made inhalation of smoke inevitable. I doubt that this accidental exposure to smoke carried as much risk as the modern habit of smoking cigarettes. Tobacco usage undeniably contributes to deaths due to heart disease, stroke and cancer. All thinking people are aware of the risk to general health, but not everyone recognizes that smoking during pregnancy carries a risk to babies. Mothers who smoke have smaller babies than nonsmoking mothers, and this growth retardation extends beyond pregnancy. School performance also suffers in smokers' children, who tend to have lower IQs and a greater incidence of attention deficit disorder than children of mothers that do not smoke.

> **Tobacco woe**
>
> *Smoking carries more risks for women than just lung cancer and ·heart disease. It leads directly to lowered fertility, miscarriage and stillbirth. Smokers suffer from more complications of pregnancy, including ectopic pregnancy, and their infants are at greater risk of low birth weight and sudden infant death syndrome.*

The breast: a nutritional treasure trove

Throughout her pregnancy Sal had little leisure time. She was expected to keep up with the activities of the other women until just hours before labor pains began. Her two sisters comforted her as the painful contractions came closer together. Seconds after the baby emerged from the birth canal, it had a strong cry, and a vigorous pink wave flowed outward to the tips of her fingers and toes. As she had watched other women do, Sal put newborn Sally to the breast several times while her womb was still contracting. In the first few hours her breasts yielded only a little fluid, and it was darker and thicker than the watery, bluish milk she had seen in other mothers. But by the third day she felt their engorgement and noticed that the milk was changing. Her infant suckled vigorously and frequently; she knew that she had introduced a healthy member to her band.

The first milk Sal's baby ingested was *colostrum*, which has more protein than later milk due to its high content of antibodies. After birth, a normal baby's immune system forms protective antibodies in response to an encounter with foreign proteins or certain kinds of complex sugars, such as those we find in disease-producing bacteria. The infant in the womb is not exposed to germs, and therefore has not developed such protection. In the days and weeks after birth, potentially life-threatening viruses and bacteria will enter the newborn's body. Like every human coming into the world, Sally was immunologically naïve: she had no antibody against these invaders. Fortunately for her, Sal's milk, especially the early colostrum, contained abundant protective antibodies. In the course of evolutionary history, women who could provide their infants with preformed protection against the most frequently encountered germs extended the species. It was once thought that the protection a mother confers to her infant lasted a few months, perhaps as long as a year. We now know that it lasts for several years past the time of weaning. The longer the period of breastfeeding, the later in life this protection extends. The components of breastmilk that protect the infant from infection gradually diminish as the child's own immune mechanisms start to develop.

Medical advances that have enabled the survival of babies weighing barely a pound have produced a pool of patients who are subject to threats that didn't exist a few generations ago. Necrotizing enterocolitis (NEC) is a devastating disorder of premature infants in which portions of the small intestine become inflamed and die. No one is certain of the cause, but it affects up to 8 percent of infants that are admitted to neonatal intensive care units. It almost never occurs in infants receiving breastmilk.

Mothers who do not put their infants to the breast during the first few days of life deprive them of a unique benefit: protection from the effects of the stress that babies encounter during the birth process. The very first drops of milk contain beta-endorphins, natural hormones that alleviate pain and the effects of stress. While undergoing the rhythmic pains of a normal labor, mothers produce these beta- endorphins and pass them into breastmilk. Women who undergo Caesarean section make less of this hormone.

It's impossible to overestimate the value of breastfeeding, but only one-third of infants in the United States are breastfed for as long as three months. Breastmilk is species-specific. That is, it contains *bioactive* factors — living cells, immune substances, hormones and growth factors that are specifically designed for human infants. The milk of one species of animal cannot fully satisfy all the requirements of the young of another species. Cow's milk is an inadequate source even of macronutrients (protein, fat and carbohydrate) for newborn humans. Babies rarely develop allergies to the proteins in their mother's milk; allergy to cow's milk protein occurs in 2 to 3 percent of infants and toddlers. Cow's milk fat doesn't contain the omega-3 fatty acids that are important for the development of the infant eye and brain. Breastmilk provides approximately three times the minimum amount of DHA required during the first few months of life.

Breastfeeding and omega-3 fatty acids may also have a role in the acquisition of type 1 diabetes mellitus. In reviewing the records of children born during the 1960s and 1970s, investigators found that in those countries where the rate of breastfeeding was lowest, the incidence of type 1 diabetes in childhood was the highest. Norwegian scientists observed that omega-3 fatty acids taken during pregnancy might protect the offspring from developing type 1 diabetes. That is the disease that typically occurs in childhood, and that can only be controlled with the daily, lifelong administration of insulin. Type 1 diabetes is definitely determined by genetic factors to some degree, but external influences, possibly certain types of viral infection, also play a role. Omega-3 fatty acids may modify these nongenetic factors by reducing the inflammatory process that leads to destruction of insulin-producing cells. Sal didn't have access to cod liver oil, or to any other processed oil, but she ate many foods that had an adequate content of these important fatty acids and their precursors. If her band traveled along coastal areas she may have eaten fish, with its high content of omega-3 fatty acids. This would be consistent with the report I have just cited, which points out that those Norwegian municipalities where fisheries are located have a statistically significant lower incidence of type 1 diabetes.

There are protective complex sugars (oligosaccharides) in breastmilk that block the attachment of harmful bacteria to the intestinal cells of the infant. They are not present in cow's milk. Carotenoids are important antioxidants and are only available to humans in fruits and vegetables or in breastmilk. Cow's milk contains fewer than breastmilk, in both quantity and quality.

Factors in breastmilk that are not found in cow's milk

DHA, an omega-3 fatty acid
Immunoglobulins (antibodies)
Certain gangliosides, important in brain development
Carotenoids, which are antioxidants
Choline, an amino acid important for brain and nerve development
Live cells that contribute to immune function
Endorphins, pain-suppressing hormones
Complex oligosaccharides, sugars that inhibit bacterial infection
Lysozyme, an enzyme that destroys bacteria
Nucleotides, substances that enhance repair of the intestinal lining
Digestive enzymes

Physicians have known for more than 100 years that mother's milk contains living cells. This is not an evolutionary accident. Some of these cells prepare the infant's immune system to respond more vigorously to naturally occurring germs. A faster immune response in the Stone Age allowed those infants to produce protective antibody to invading microorganisms more speedily, enhancing their chances of survival. In an environment in which infection was a leading cause of death, especially in infancy, the advantages for continued existence of the species were enormous.

Because of this transfer of live cells in breastmilk, infants develop a tolerance to maternal cells. As a result, a kidney that is transplanted later in life from mother to child has a better chance of survival.

Every drop of infant formula is identical to every other. The composition of human milk changes over time in accordance with the needs of the infant. *Nelson's Textbook of Pediatrics* lists 88 factors and characteristics of breastmilk that vary over time according to the age of the infant. There are sound biological reasons why the components of breastmilk (which actually number in the thousands, not just 88) change every few days from the first day until weaning is complete. For instance, the content of gangliosides, critical components of the brain and nervous system, varies markedly from colostrum to later human milk. It is higher in breastmilk than in cow's milk or commercial formula. Proteins are orders of magnitude more complex than fats or carbohydrates, and vary tremendously from one species to another. Factors in colostrum appear to regulate the manufacture of proteins. These factors are unique to human infants and are obviously lacking in commercial formulas.

This exquisite interaction between mother and infant is almost impossible to comprehend. Nature even provides for the infant that is born ahead of schedule. Omega-3 fatty acids such as DHA pass to the growing fetus in large amounts during the last two months of pregnancy. This is when growth of the brain and eye demands a large supply of omega-3 fatty acids. How does this affect the infant who is born several weeks too early? The breastmilk of the mother who delivers prematurely has a higher fatty acid content than that of mothers who carry their infants a full 9 months, and so delivers a compensatory load of these crucial components to her child. This ensures that the infant who arrives early will function normally, and will contribute to survival of the species.

Physicians refer to the mother-infant couple as a dyad. This implies that they function as a biological unit. One particular phenomenon shows how intricate this relationship is. If a woman has low body fat stores, which was not uncommon among prehistoric people, she will produce breastmilk with a lower fat content. As if to compensate, the infant will prolong its suckling.

Breastfeeding has both immediate and long-term benefits for the mother. In the period immediately following delivery, the infant's nursing stimulates contraction of the uterus and reduces blood loss. This would have been an enormous survival benefit during the Stone Age. Women who breastfeed have a lower incidence of breast cancer during the years prior to menopause, and the longer the period of breastfeeding, the lower the risk.

Physicians recognized the protective effects of breastfeeding many years ago, before antibiotics changed the course of childhood infections. Modern medicine now contends with chronic disease, most of which is caused by a lifestyle that is discordant with our genetic makeup. Just as breastfeeding can influence resistance to microbes during the first decade of life, it can influence noninfectious diseases during the last.

In susceptible individuals, obesity and type 2 diabetes are closely linked. Breastfed infants seem to be less likely to become obese later in childhood. It may be a leap to conjecture that breastfed babies, being less likely to become obese, are less likely to develop type 2 diabetes later in life, but that is what occurs among the Pima Indians of the American southwest (Chapter Five). Breastfeeding may even modify the chances of heart disease late in life. Cholesterol levels in adults are lower in those who were breastfed as infants.

Asthma is a major disease of childhood, one that has more than doubled in some population groups in a single generation. In spite of its frequency, asthma is one of the least understood diseases in both children and adults. Exposure to tobacco smoke is one factor. Studies on children in Australia suggest that exclusive breastfeeding for at least 4 months lessens the likelihood that a child will develop asthma.

Given a healthy baby, most mothers are next concerned about their child's intelligence. It was probably the same during the Stone Age. Does breastfeeding make a difference? It does, especially in those parts of the world where alternatives to breastfeeding are substandard. Several studies have suggested that IQ and scholastic achievement are better among children who are breastfed for at least 6 months. The differences were not great, but they included standard tests of intelligence, reading ability and mathematics, as well as teacher evaluations. In Denmark, where authorities keep careful and detailed records on breastfeeding, adults who were breastfed scored significantly better on two different intelligence tests. Among very premature infants there is a significant positive association between feeding of human milk and verbal IQ. Perhaps that's because those early arrivals that are formula-fed miss out on the late-pregnancy delivery of omega-3 fatty acids, and receive no replacement.

One advantage of breastfeeding may be related to its content of docosahexaenoic acid (DHA) and arachidonic acid (AA). When these fatty acids were added to infant formula, some measures of visual and brain development were significantly higher than those of infants fed standard formula.

Hypertension is one of the epidemic chronic diseases of our time, affecting more than half the population over the age of 40. Researchers have suspected that infants who were breastfed have lower blood pressure later in life. A confirmatory study comes from England, where researchers followed breastfed premature infants until their early teens. These children had lower blood pressures than their nursery mates who were formula-fed.

After breastfeeding

During my years in pediatric practice, the eagerness mothers showed in giving their babies solid foods often amused me. Some mothers added cereal to the bottle of formula. They insisted that this helped the infant (and the parents) to sleep through the night, but careful studies show that this is not true. By the time the infant is 2 ½ months of age the parental frustration factor reaches its peak. This is about the time when infants will sleep through the night if their parents are able to judiciously ignore their crying. Few mothers can resist the urge to start solid feeding by the third month, although the American Academy of Pediatrics recommends six months of exclusive breastfeeding.

Sal probably nursed Sally for more than a year, possibly for several years. The baby's first solids consisted of food that had been chewed by her mother (premastication), a practice that today's mothers find unacceptable, or worse. Why bother when there is plenty of cereal, fruit, vegetables, meat and mixed dinners in convenient glass jars at the supermarket? Sal had little choice. Pottery vessels were unknown until at least a few thousand years before the Agricultural Revolution. Before

Advocates of breastfeeding maintain that nursing infants should be fed whenever they signal their hunger by crying. That is consistent with infant feeding practices among hunter-gatherers, and it is certain to have been the norm prior to the advent of artificial, i.e., cow's milk or formula, feeding. The expectation of modern parents that infants should sleep through the night within a few weeks after birth is not normal for our species.

then, gourds, animal skins, shells or hollowed wood served in their place, and feeding utensils were far, far in the future. When Sal prechewed her baby's first solid food she gave her two benefits. First, the child enjoyed almost as wide a variety of foods as her mother did. Second, Sal added enzymes from her own saliva to this food. In the multimillennia before the use of fire, this probably had some nutritional advantage. Cooking releases nutrients in many foods, breaking down fiber and releasing carbohydrates and protein. Chewing and salivary enzymes do the same; they are an important part of the digestive process at all ages beyond infancy. Enzymes in the intestine work better when we chew food thoroughly because it presents a larger surface area on which they can act. Sally's infantile digestive system could therefore tolerate foods that she might otherwise not absorb well, or that might cause digestive disturbances.

Babies are ready for transitional foods well before the first birthday. How parents accommodate their children's desire for solid foods can have a major impact on their future health. There are three important goals of childhood feeding that can reverse the maladaptive trends that prevail today: first, to increase children's intake of fruits and vegetables; second, to decrease the intake of energy-dense fats and sugars; third, to avoid overeating in general.

It will be difficult to attain these goals as long as publications that originate from the United States Department of Agriculture and the National Cancer Institute refer to bread, meat, milk, cheese, white potatoes, ready-to-eat-cereal, pasta, rice and grains as nutritious staples. Except for meat, not a single one of these foods was present during the thousands of millennia during which our body chemistry developed. That most of us tolerate them without any overt or immediate problems overlooks the fact that we have far more nutritious staples available that are more compatible with our genetic endowment. I am not arguing for elimination of grain- and dairy product-based foods, but only intend to emphasize the value of a diet high in fruits and vegetables. Unless we lead children to this pattern at a very early age, they will be at high risk of chronic diseases that have already reached epidemic proportions in this country.

A mother's influence on the later food preferences of her child begins in the first few days of its life if she breastfeeds. Formula-fed infants accept new foods less readily than those who are breastfed. It may be due to the fact that formula comes in only one flavor, while the taste of breastmilk reflects the mother's intake. Surprisingly, infants stay attached to the nipple longer if breastmilk has been flavored with vanilla or garlic than if the mother has been on a bland diet. During my practice years I counseled mothers to avoid spices, garlic and onions, having been taught that these foods, passing through the breast, might cause colicky pain in infants. We now know that that is simply not true. In fact, infants whose mothers eat garlic prior to breastfeeding will stay on the breast even longer. We do know that there is a subset of infants who will have less colicky pain if their mother avoids cow's milk protein.

What foods the parents make available and eat themselves influence the child's developing eating habits. When fruits and vegetables are regularly available and accessible, this has a positive effect. It even extends to foods that the child initially does not like. Preschool children, watching their peers choosing and eating vegetables that they themselves don't like, gradually develop a preference for these foods. A striking example is the acquisition of taste for chili peppers. Neither humans nor animals have a natural preference for the flavor of chili, but Mexican children model the behavior they see in their families. The influence of the family on a child's food preferences is greatest with young children, and declines as they get older. Young children, as every parent knows, have a dislike for vegetables, but this gradually diminishes, especially if these foods are offered repeatedly, and if they are presented attractively. This could include colorful condiments (chopped sweet red and green pepper, yellow corn) and small amounts of flavorful sauces.

Children should be picky eaters; it's in their genes

The fact that parents influence the food preferences of younger children is rooted in evolution, and has survival benefits. Sal could not let little Sally sample whatever she wanted in her primitive environment, lest it be poisonous. She received her first solid foods from her parents. They knew that these foods were safe. Sally could therefore be expected to accept new foods only after she repeatedly saw her parents and peers partaking of these foods. Nature may have programmed us to avoid strange foods as a safety mechanism, protecting the curious toddler. Today's children may undergo the same process for the same reasons. Perhaps parents who accept this will be less frustrated at mealtimes.

Nurture without nourishment

Among the top 10 food sources of energy among children are cake, cookies, donuts, ready-to-eat cereal, soda, potato chips, popcorn, sugar, syrup and jam. Except for white potatoes (#15), not a single fruit or vegetable was among the top 29 foods in one study. An analysis of the meals of second- and fifth-grade students revealed that 40 percent of them ate no vegetables on the days studied, yet 36 percent of them ate 4 or more snack foods on those days. More than 97 percent of children consume fewer than 3 servings of vegetables per day.

Most mothers think that fruit juice is a healthy drink. It is, but much of what we now find on the supermarket shelf is not really juice, but a fruit drink. The actual fruit juice content of these beverages is often less than 10 percent, but it's almost impossible to determine that from the label. In order to make them more appealing, manufacturers intentionally make these drinks sweeter than natural juices by adding even more fructose and sorbitol. Although both of these sugars are naturally present in fruit, fructose is not absorbed as well as glucose and can cause chronic diarrhea and abdominal pain. When sorbitol is present it worsens the already poor absorption of fructose. Fruit juice has little of the fiber, pectin and other nutrients of whole fruit. Various studies confirm that as fruit juice consumption increases, milk intake decreases.

> Sam and Sal's children drank only water. Ours drink juice, fruit drinks, carbonated beverages and milk. American preschoolers are probably not much different from their British counterparts, more than half of whom do not drink plain water at all.

One of the most discouraging sights I have encountered as a pediatrician is the toddler whose teeth are no more than brown-black stumps; the surviving crowns are sometimes rotted to the gum line. I have seen scores of these babies who were tucked into bed with a bottle of juice or milk at hand. The sugar in these liquids promotes early childhood caries, massive decay that can begin within a matter of weeks. The American Academy of Pediatrics and the American Academy of Pediatric Dentistry have issued joint statements discouraging the use of juices from a bottle.

Zeroing in on the problem

There are two strong factors that influence inappropriate food preferences: parents and television.

Parents offer sweets and high-fat snacks as rewards for good behavior. Ice cream, cake and candy are associated with feasting and fun (birthdays, etc.). They sometimes withhold these foods as punishment for bad behavior, or for not eating "good" foods. Sweets and snacks then become either forbidden fruit or pleasant rewards. These preferences become stronger in adult life, sometimes resulting in binge eating.

Television, the "perverse purveyor of culture," does influence children's food preferences. Most of the advertising that is shown during children's programming is for food products, the majority of which have very low nutritional value. Children acquire preferences from those ads and do influence the parents' purchase of those foods. Years of TV viewing could hardly result in a yearning for fruits and vegetables, which only appear occasionally as cartoon characters ("Archibald Asparagus," in *Veggie Tales,* Big Idea Productions, Inc., Chicago IL).

Children have the innate capacity to regulate their energy intake and maintain balance with energy expenditure. Infants stop nursing when they are satiated. Formula-fed babies also reach satiety based on the calories their caretakers offer them. Even at 6 weeks, an infant will take more of a diluted formula than a conventional one, controlling his energy intake. However, a mother can override the regulatory ability of her infant by encouraging him to finish the bottle, even though the baby has fulfilled his caloric needs for the day.

Older children also have an efficient energy-balancing capability. If offered an energy-dense first portion of a two-course meal, they will eat less when offered a second course. The ability to self-select based on energy requirements operates for about 24 hours at a time. As in the case of formula-fed infants, parents can override this energy-balancing mechanism. A child who is rewarded for being a member of the Clean Plate Club or who is consistently encouraged to eat more will eventually rely on external cues instead of internal ones. Such parental prompts produce overweight children.

The enormous changes in family structure and parenting relationships during the past half-century confound analysis and complicate recommendations. Barely 25 percent of children live in a traditional family: original parents, married and living together. Single parents, shared custody, grandparents raising grandchildren, and day care comprise a mix of child management practices. Where once the mother alone determined her children's diet, that role is overshadowed by day care facilities. There are 21 million children in the United States under the age of 6 years; 13 million of them are in some form of childcare facility outside the home. Most children eat one or two meals, plus snacks, at day care facilities, many of which serve meals of poor quality that do not supply key nutrients, but do provide too much fat.

The obese child: undermining the future

Obesity is increasing just as dramatically among children in the United States as it is in adults. The appalling statistics are that 30 percent of children are overweight and 15 percent are obese. Even the growth charts that pediatricians use in their offices have had to be revised. At the same time, the general state of American children's nutrition is declining. We cannot overstate the dangers of childhood obesity. As many as 25 percent of obese children have abnormally high blood sugar, including those as young as 4 years of age. Sixty percent of obese children already have high blood pressure, abnormal blood fat profiles and excess insulin production. Ten percent of obese Japanese youths have blood tests that reveal abnormalities in liver function. Breathing difficulties during sleep are common in obese children. Preteen obese children have thickened arteries resembling those of lifetime smokers.

Insulin resistance is a predictor of type 2 diabetes, an expensive, lifestyle-shattering illness that is already becoming commonplace in pediatricians' offices. It has increased 10-fold in Cincinnati since 1982. The Centers for Disease Control, in what should have been a wake-up call to the nation, reported in 2003 that of children born in the year 2000, more than one-third would develop diabetes during their lifetime. Among Latino girls the expected number is 53 percent, and African-American girls are not far behind at 49 percent. Those of us who have been tracking this problem for years are strongly of the opinion that these figures are underestimates.

As children spend more time engaged in watching television, playing video games and acquiring computer skills, the upward trend in childhood obesity and the inevitable climb in the rate of adult cardiovascular diseases and diabetes will continue. We don't have to wait until another generation of TV-watching children grows up. We already know that children who watch television four or more hours each day are fatter than those who watch it less than two hours a day.

The social consequences of obesity are more subtle than its medical complications, especially among women. Persons who are overweight have lower incomes and are more likely to live below the poverty line than those of normal weight. They are also less likely to marry, and spend fewer years in school.

Although obesity is not linked to a high risk of psychological problems, the fear of obesity is. This extends to family members, who may be reluctant to discuss weight problems with a child because they are afraid that she will diet excessively, and perhaps develop anorexia nervosa or bulimia. Anorexia nervosa is a disorder in which the young person, usually female, has a distorted perception of her body. She may have an intense fear of becoming obese, and considers herself too fat even when she is obviously underweight. Bulimia may be even more common, and consists of binge eating followed either by self-induced vomiting, the use of laxatives or rigorous fasting. Persons with bulimia may have normal weight, or may even be slightly obese, and the problem is more difficult to recognize.

If a preschool child is overweight it does not necessarily indicate that he or she will be overweight in adult life. However, about half of overweight preschoolers do become overweight adults. Fifty percent is not a small number, and this is clearly the age at which we must begin. Infants should not be coaxed to take the last ounce from the bottle. You can trust their appetite. The same is true of toddlers. Parents should not force them to eat everything that is set before them. They are natural "grazers" at this age and will take in enough calories if they have access to food. However, parents should be careful to avoid the path of least resistance: sugary snacks and fruit juices. We should guide children toward having fresh fruit for dessert, in the Italian style.

When parents overcontrol their children's eating pattern, it promotes eating more of the restricted foods, whereas providing open access to healthy foods encourages eating those foods. Guiding a child toward healthy foods is impossible when junk food is constantly available at home.

The school years

When children enter school they have access to a large selection of fat- and sugar-laden snack foods, as well as nutrient-null soft drinks. It isn't advisable for parents to demonize these unhealthy foods; it can only make the child want more of them. But if the home environment has matter-of-factly presented wholesome choices to the child on a daily basis, occasional junk food forays with their peers will be less harmful. Some school cafeterias provide excellent meals, but in a system that regards a packet of catsup as a vegetable serving and where pizza is available every day, that's probably not the norm. Students also have access to high-fat and high-sugar snacks at vending machines and school stores. When they provide wholesome meals at home, parents can not only fill a nutritional void, but also instill good health habits by example.

The adolescent years are the perfect time to encourage physical activity by participation in sports programs, both in and out of school, taking advantage of adolescents' energy and competitiveness. Neither parents nor school authorities are making the best use of this opportunity. Physical activity of children shows a steady decline during the school years, especially among girls. By positively encouraging physical activity during childhood and adolescence, parents, physicians and educators can lead young people into a lifestyle pattern that will yield immense health benefits for several decades. Parents may underestimate their influence in this matter. They should be aware that children whose mothers and fathers lead physically active lives are 6 times as likely to be active than children whose parents are inactive.

We tend to regard obesity as a matter of overeating, but in fact, it is really a matter of underexercise. An energy intake of 5,000 calories a day should certainly lead to obesity if it is maintained for a long period, but Arctic explorers typically take in this much during their journeys, and sometimes return weighing less than when they started. More than one mother has watched a loaf of bread and a half-gallon of milk disappear along with a pound of sandwich meat when her teenage son brings a couple of friends home after a ballgame. She recognizes that this is normal eating behavior for the age and circumstance. Teenagers, just like Arctic explores, use up the calories they take in. They don't gain weight until they decrease their physical activity.

With adolescence, of course, comes puberty, and dietary factors play a role here as well. As obesity has drawn the attention of researchers in many fields, some have observed that overweight girls enter puberty earlier than girls of normal weight. They must acquire a certain amount of fat for the reproductive process to be set in motion. This seems to be regulated by a hormone known as leptin.

Leptin is formed in fat cells. As the amount of fat tissue increases, so does the leptin level. According to the leptin theory, it acts as part of a feedback mechanism that regulates appetite. Scientists, basing their theory on studies in animals, hoped initially that a deficiency of leptin would explain why humans become obese, but they found that a system that operates in mice does not always operate the same way in humans. Leptin levels are low during childhood and increase at the onset of puberty. This suggests that it signals the brain that fat levels are adequate and it is safe for pregnancy to occur. The actual picture is not nearly as simple as I have painted it, but it may help to explain why adolescents start puberty earlier than they did in decades past.

How can modern parents help their children to develop lifelong healthy eating habits and stop the upward spiral of obesity and diabetes? One answer may be fiber. As I have mentioned in earlier chapters, the eating pattern for which our bodies are designed predates even Sam and Sal, the examples of our Stone Age ancestors of 50,000 years ago.

Their fiber intake was about 10 times ours, and came from fruits and vegetables. We don't need to — and probably could not — eat that much in order to gain its benefits: lower calorie intake while feeling satiated, reduced risk of type 2 diabetes, stroke and heart disease, and a reduced risk of colon and other types of cancer. A moderately high fiber intake will result in less weight gain in young persons, even if their fat intake is relatively high as a percentage of total daily calories.

We can easily attain a fiber intake of 20 grams or more per day by using the government guidelines of 5 fruits and 4 vegetables per day. The shopping suggestions I proposed in Chapter Six and the feeding strategies listed earlier in this chapter are key elements: don't buy what you don't want your children to eat, make fruits and vegetables readily available for grazing, and set the example by not indulging in calorie-laden sweets and fats.

Is this easy? Not for families whose children already have well-established eating habits. It's harder still for parents who themselves are overweight. But the rewards are enormous in terms of enhanced health, greater self-esteem, better career opportunities, safer childbirth and lower risk of eating disorders. In Chapter Nine I will outline reasonable and attainable approaches to Rediscovering Your Genetic Pathway, so that you and your family will:

* Feel better
* Look better
* Be safer
* Be stronger
* Not be hungry
* Not have to count calories
* Save money

Nine

Rediscover your genetic pathway

Most people have a termite lifestyle.
You can't see the damage until something collapses.

OTHER FORMS OF life follow their genetic pathways under the influence of environmental elements over which they have no control, like leaves that have fallen into a roiling stream. We are doing what no other species, among millions on the planet, has ever done. We are creating new pathways and overriding our gene structure. Sooner than many people think, we will be able to modify our genes, repair their defective elements and overcome perceived shortcomings. To a great extent, and sometimes at a high price, we have overcome natural enemies, from saber-toothed tigers to smallpox viruses. We have created new ones — tobacco smoke and toxic smog. Even earth's remaining hunter-gatherers, those dwindling descendents of Sam and Sal, are acquiring modern maladies.

The ancestors of Sam and Sal were simple creatures, yet they survived, thrived and multiplied in a world of predators and primitive conditions. They were, after all, part of the food chain, and not necessarily at the top of it. Thomas Hobbes described their lives as "nasty, brutish and short." I can't help but wonder if these same lives would have been "serene, humane and long" if they only had decent plumbing! In the absence of other human predators, it is safe homes, clean water and an adequate food supply that allow us to escape most of the misery that life throws our way. Much credit surely is due to medical science but civilization could have advanced without many of its achievements, and longevity is not a recent phenomenon. The Greek playwright Sophocles lived to 90 years, and Michelangelo to 89, long before the discovery of antibiotics, anesthesia and antihypertensive drugs.

> Old age and senility are not synon-ymous. When a reporter asked Frenchwoman Jeanne Calment, the then-oldest living human, what she thought the rest of her life would be like, she replied, "Short. Very short." She lived to celebrate her 122nd birthday.

Albert Szent-Gyorgi, the renowned scientist of the early twentieth century, observed, "for every complex problem, there is a simple, easy to understand, incorrect answer." At the risk of adding my name to the list of those who have confirmed the wisdom of that statement, I will submit my own "simple, easy to understand" proposals. Sam and Sal will guide us along the path to health, vigor and longevity, and modern science will buttress with authority what Sam and Sal discovered by accident. I'll offer some general princi-ples, describe how they can be applied in daily life, and list various ways by which you can implement these suggestions.

Except in the case of injury or acute, severe infection, there is usually a period of declining health and vigor that precedes death. One of the goals of this book is to make that period of decline a short one, and to delay the time of onset. If we follow the examples of our Stone Age ancestors we can alleviate or postpone chronic, nonfatal diseases such as osteoarthritis, and disorders of vision and hearing. Thus we can provide a *compression of morbidity*, shorten-ing that period between disability and death.

Health, vigor and longevity result from sensible lifestyle choices. These are more important than ever, because opportunities to make poor ones besiege us. Three simple factors underlie the pathway to good health: appropriate physical activity, proper food choices and management of stress.

That is not to say that we can always be in command of our health. How about the perils we can't avoid? Environmental hazards, such as smog and pollution, and motor vehicle accidents, account for an estimated 100,000 deaths per year. They are devastating to the individuals who suffer from them, yet they are lesser factors in our overall survival. In contrast, heart disease alone causes 7 times as many deaths per year as accidents, and cancer almost 6 times as many. A healthy body can tolerate toxins better than an unhealthy one. Injuries heal faster in a well person, and a competent immune system can better impede secondary infection. The most serious threats to our health and well-being are the ones we can avoid.

Physical activity

It is not exaggerating to say that if all humans were as physically active as Sam and Sal were, more than half the premature deaths due to heart disease, stroke and diabetes would not occur. In fact, even moderate activity brings significant improvement in death rates from these diseases. In the case of women with type 2 diabetes, exercise for one hour or more per day can lower the heart disease risk by almost half — 45 percent. More evidence is accumulating that regular exercise can even lower the risk of breast cancer.

It's not just our muscles that benefit from regular activity, but our brains. In a study of almost 6,000 otherwise healthy women, those who kept active by walking, gardening or doing similar nonstrenuous activities were nearly 30 percent less likely to show mental decline than those who were least active. As I noted in Chapter Four, our genetic makeup requires that we exercise regularly. That means almost every day. It does not mean that the exercise must be intense or last all day. A little reflection on the day-to-day pattern of activity of our Stone Age ancestors, or even their modern-day hunter-gatherer counterparts, shows that performing regular "huthold" chores and the acquisition of food accounted for most of their action. The typical American would have to walk an additional 12 miles a day to match the activity level of present-day hunter-gatherers, but we can do far less and still reap major benefits.

Although we can maintain our fitness level in three or four sessions of resistance exercise, and by walking for 30 or 40 minutes three or four times a week, we can also gain health benefits if we make slight alterations in how we go about our daily routine. I have called these "Minirobics™." They can partly substitute for the 30 to 60 minutes of exercise a day we ought to do. Make these activities part of your regular routine.

Minirobics™: stealth exercise

You don't have to have special shoes or clothing, or go to the gym to get the benefits of exercise and increase your muscle tone. There are lots of opportunities around us every day for increased physical activity. Some of these motions seem to involve so few calories that it wouldn't seem to make any difference, but all activity is beneficial if it keeps muscles moving. Remember that if you use only 10 calories a day more than you take in, you'll lose about one pound of fat per year. Between the ages of 25 and 55 the average American gains about one pound a year, what I referred to earlier as creeping obesity.

Do you ever take a down elevator? If you're only going a couple of floors it might be faster to take the stairs. If you're going up a flight or two, why not walk? All those calories count, all activity improves muscle tone, and every breath deeper than those you take at rest improves your oxygen-carrying capacity.

Where do you park when you go shopping? Most of us drive around the lot a couple of times, looking for the closest spot. I used to do that, too. Now I park at the farthest corner, where my car has less chance of being dented by another car's door.

I used to look for the closest parking space when I went to the fitness center. The fitness center! Now I park at the other end of the lot, where I never have to jockey for space. I also get part of my warm-up done by the time I reach the front door of the center. On the way back I can cool down, which is important after a moderate workout.

Parking at a distance has another benefit: I have never lost my car. This works just as well in any business location.

Have you ever moved your car from one parking space to another at the shopping center if you have to visit two stores? Park in the middle of the lot and get a little more exercise. You'll burn more calories and less gas.

The stairway in your home gives you the same exercise as a stair-climbing machine. The extra trips up and down are no longer a nuisance. They are helping you to maintain your fitness.

If you have several things to carry from one place to another, why not do it in two trips instead of one? There's less chance of dropping something.

If you mow your lawn, get a push-type mower. It's cheaper, safer, hardly ever breaks down, and never runs out of gas. You also won't have potentially dangerous gasoline in your garage.

Yard work and gardening are among the best forms of physical activity, because they are also stress-relieving.

How often do you go to the supermarket? Why not go two or three times a week instead of one? Carry a couple of bags out of the store instead of pushing a wagonload. Your heart, lungs and legs will be a little stronger, and your veggies will be a little fresher.

If you push a vacuum cleaner around the house every couple of days instead of once a week, you'll have a cleaner, less dusty house, as well as stronger arms and shoulders.

Hide the TV remote.

Walk your child to the bus stop instead of driving her there.

Going to the bank? Go around the drive-through window, park across the street or at the far end of the parking lot, and walk to the lobby.

If you work at a computer all day, put the phone where you have to get up to reach it. That also reduces computer fatigue.

Get a dog and let it take you for a walk every day.

At work, go to the rest room that's farthest away, not the closest one.

At the kids' ballgames, pace the sidelines instead of sitting in the stands.

Keep a pair of comfortable walking shoes in your car. They'll give you inspiration to use them, and it could become a habit.

Wash your car by hand every week instead of sitting in it as it goes through the car wash. You can do the average-sized vehicle in about 30 minutes, and you'll save about $500 a year.

Make it a priority to play catch, football, jump rope or hit golf balls with a child or grandchild every single week. It's far more than just exercise. For you it's good conditioning. For them, it will add to their storehouse of cherished memories.

The exercise pathway

First, understand that your body is designed for more intense physical activity than the average person performs, and that failure to keep up with nature's requirements will lead directly and inevitably to the conditions that we usually blame on aging — overweight, arthritis, heart disease, diabetes and a lack of energy.

Second, it takes only 30 to 60 minutes a day, most days of the week, to maintain good physical condition. Moderate intensity is all that's required, and it doesn't have to be done all at one time. Most centenarians have never lifted weights or jogged, but they are probably very familiar with the daily activities I described above.

There are guidelines for resistance-type exercises in Appendix 2, and for selecting equipment in Appendix 1. If you follow these guidelines, use light weights, and walk at a moderate pace at least three times a week, you'll accomplish more than 90 percent of the population, and you'll be among the 10 percent who look better and who feel better all the time.

Proper food choices

It's never easy to make wholesale changes in dietary patterns, and the bigger your family, the more likely it is that someone will vigorously oppose rocking the boat. Although it doesn't have to be done all at once, making large changes is actually easier than a piecemeal approach. One reason is that major substitutions, such as switching from the usual baked goods to those made only with whole wheat, or eliminating fried foods from the household menu, show a genuine commitment, not a flimsy one. That sends a signal to everyone that you're serious, and reinforces your own belief.

A second reason is that you will feel better when you make major changes, but won't notice much improvement with minor ones. As an example, when you add more vegetables to the regular menu and have plenty of fruit available for snacks instead of junk food, you'll avoid feelings of hunger and the drowsiness that occurs after a spike and fall in blood sugar. It only takes a few days to notice the difference.

You have probably read articles or books whose authors advocate avoiding the "great white toxins": white flour, white rice, white sugar, white milk and salt. The label is a little extreme, but the concept is not. Sam and Sal had no access to any of them. If all these foods were to disappear from our world overnight, no one's health would suffer. Apart from energy-supplying carbohydrates, the first three are nutrient-null, except for what food manufacturers restore artificially. Whole-wheat flour and brown rice are more nutritious and flavorful than their white counterparts. Artificial sweeteners have already replaced sugar in many foods, but not everyone would agree that they are safe substitutes. Contrary to the commercial, hardly anyone needs milk. Despite its shortcomings however, cow's milk is difficult to replace for children under the age of two years, who need it as a source of calcium, protein and fat. As an idealist-pediatrician I yearn for the Utopia in which all children are breastfed for 24 months.

There is a diet that is delicious, nutritious and economical. Hundreds of millions of people already adhere to it. Physicians around the world recommend it. Americans have modified it. It is the Mediterranean diet.

The Mediterranean diet: a bridge from the Stone Age to today

The Mediterranean Sea bathes the beaches of 19 nations. There is an enormous variation in the native diets of these countries. If you were to travel from Spain to Syria, from Italy to Egypt, you'd quickly notice the differences. Which one takes ownership of the true Mediterranean diet?

A half-century ago, Ancel Keys and other public health specialists observed that the people of Crete had adult life expectancies that were among the highest in the world. The rates of cancer, coronary artery disease and some other diet-related diseases were among the lowest anywhere. It is that island whose nutritional norms Dr. Keys carefully measured and chronicled. Later studies focused on Italy, Greece and other Mediterranean countries, hence the name. Strictly speaking, it is the 1960s version of that dietary pattern on the island of Crete to which we properly apply the name Mediterranean diet. Some authors use the diet of Southern Italy as a prototype, and it is emerging as the "gold standard of heart disease prevention." But don't look for the true Mediterranean diet at your local pizza parlor or Italian restaurant.

Pasta, prosciutto and provolone; feta, pita and baclava. They have a nice Mediterranean ring, but these are not the main, or even common, constituents of the diet of that name. On the island of Crete and in southern Italy in the 1960s, coarse bread (without butter or margarine), cereals and potatoes comprised the greatest sources of energy. Vegetables, beans, fruits and nuts made up most of the remainder. Although there has been a drift toward more meat and saturated fat, the eating pattern of most southern Italians still retains most of the characteristics that Keys and his colleagues described.

One of the myths of the Mediterranean diet is that it is high in dairy products, but that is so only in northern Italy. The southern coastal areas lacked refrigeration until relatively recently, which made it impossible to keep whole milk, butter or cream. Yogurt and cheese are the representative dairy components of the region. The large amounts of cheese in a single serving of our pizza, ravioli or manicotti would last a Cretan family for days. They would serve it in small amounts, as a garnish, not as a main course. Red meat is not regular fare in Mediterranean countries, especially in Crete, where the average intake is a little more than one-half ounce per day. They also eat only small or moderate amounts of poultry. The average intake of eggs is less than 4 per week, and that includes those that are used in the preparation of other dishes.

One would imagine that countries that together enjoy several thousand miles of coastline would have a high per capita intake of fish, but that is only true of Spain and Portugal. (The latter borders on the Atlantic, not the Mediterranean.) Those who live in Crete and Italy eat fish in low to moderate amounts, and it is not a

> *Dr. Keys described the cardiac gradient of Italy. The incidence of heart disease increased as one moved north from the toe of the peninsula to its borders with Austria, France and Switzerland. People in the north of Italy consume far more animal products than those in the south, less fish, and far fewer plant foods.*

daily food item. They do, however, eat more fish than Americans do. Seafood constitutes an important source of omega-3 fatty acids, which I described in previous chapters. Those who live along the Mediterranean coast eat about 7 ounces a week, an amount that provides adequate essential fatty acids for good health.

The cultural ascent of modern humans, represented in this book by Sam and Sal, took place largely in the Mediterranean basin, first in the eastern areas, then to the west and north. Before they developed tools, they subsisted on vegetables, fruits, roots and nuts. Those foods still form the core of the Mediterranean diet, and most of them are locally grown, varying by season. This generous intake of plant foods may be one of the reasons why nutritionists regard the Mediterranean diet so highly. Its ample fiber content has been correlated with a lower rate of coronary artery disease and colon cancer, the high folic acid level with fewer congenital defects of the brain and spinal cord, and its variety of antioxidants with a low incidence of cataracts and other illnesses. The small bands of prehistoric people who wandered along the coast ate no grain-based foods, and had a greater intake of meat than those who dwell there now, but the remainder of their diet was very similar to that of the vigorous villagers of Crete and its neighbors, who still eat a predominately Stone Age diet.

Vegetables, legumes and fruits contain more than 4,000 micronutrients in addition to the well-known antioxidants such as vitamins C and E, selenium and beta-carotene. This plethora of phytonutrients includes quercetin, lutein, kaempferol, indoles, dithiolthiones, allium compounds, limonene, phenols, and isoflavones such as genistein and daidzein. Not all of them are present in all species of plants, but each one is likely to play some role in human nutrition. For this reason, nutritionists agree that we should partake of a large variety of plant foods.

Olive oil has been the principal source of fat in the Mediterranean region for thousands of years. It is almost the only source (95 percent) of added fat in southern Italy. Unlike the dairy fats that are a major portion of the diet in northern Italy and other European countries, olive oil has little saturated fat. The fatty acids it does contain are those that are related to heart health, and help to prevent the untimely formation of blood clots. There is very little omega-3 fatty acid in olive oil, but there are other, ample sources of these in the Mediterranean diet, including fish and vegetables. The meat and eggs of free-roaming poultry also contain more omega-3 fatty acids that those of their grain-fed counterparts in the United States.

Perhaps the secret of the Mediterranean diet is right under our noses, and food is only a small part of it. Almost the only common factors

> The high levels of monounsaturated fatty acids in olive oil decrease LDL (bad) cholesterol and increase HDL (good) cholesterol. Other chemicals protect the lining of blood vessels. It contains a variety of phytochemicals, including those that appear to lower the risk of several types of cancer. Olive oil also reduces the risk of gallstones by enhancing gallbladder emptying.

among the millions who inhabit the shores of the Mediterranean are the sea that gives the region its name, and a high level of physical activity. Obesity and its consequences are uncommon among these peoples because their energy expenditure matches their intake. They are not wealthy, and do not enjoy the culinary excesses of those that are. That was especially true in the post-World War II period when Keys and his colleagues conducted their studies in Crete and other European countries. The Cretan culture was poor and unmechanized — and healthy. Keys found that the life expectancy of Greek males in 1960 was the highest in any population reported during that period, and premature mortality from heart disease was 90 percent lower than that for American males. Yet, Leland Allbaugh, an epidemiologist who conducted similar studies at about the same time, quoted one of his subjects: "We are hungry most of the time." Could that be a clue?

It is more than 60 years since researchers observed that low-calorie, high-nutritive diets were associated with dramatic increases in longevity in laboratory animals. The theory is probably valid, and there are some suggestions that well-controlled underfeeding has real benefits in humans. Calorie restriction does not require a crash diet. It is a deliberate, slow process. Proponents of the method point out that it takes several years to reach a weight that is about 20 percent below the norm for height.

There are some serious, well-disciplined practitioners of this method, including Dr. Roy Walford, Professor of Pathology at University of California at Los Angeles Medical School. Unfortunately, no matter how many years it may add to one's life, the spartan regimen is not a very attractive trade-off for most people. Nor, in addition, is the fragile-appearing physique that it imparts. If you can tolerate feeling cold much of the time and having little sex drive in order to perhaps live 20 or 30 years longer than most humans, you might be a candidate for calorie restriction.

Sam and Sal may well have had some contemporaries who unintentionally lived the calorie-restricted lifestyle for long periods. As long as the intake of essential minerals and micronutrients is adequate, being a little hungry much of the time is not harmful. The Crete illustration is a good example. We find another in Okinawans, whose calorie intake is far below other Japanese. They have one of the lowest rates of heart disease in the world, the longest lifespan of any group, and a higher percentage of centenarians than any recorded population.

Wine

"Wine can be considered with good reason as the most healthful and most hygienic of all beverages." – Louis Pasteur

If wine drinkers need any justification for their enjoyment of wine, science has come to their rescue. Medical researchers have long been aware that those who drink wine have a lower risk of heart attacks than those who do not, and they are finally unraveling the mystery. Some phytonutrients in wine increase HDL (good) cholesterol and lower the heart-damaging effects of LDL (bad) cholesterol. Other components lower total cholesterol and limit the damage that free radicals do to the lining of blood vessels. A small study from Australia suggests that moderate wine intake and lower homocysteine levels may be related, but a healthy intake of leafy green vegetables will also reduce homocysteine levels.

It's not only the heart that might benefit from the hundreds of phenols, flavonoids, saponins and other ingredients of wine. They also reduce the likelihood that we will develop type 2 diabetes or Alzheimer's disease, and they protect the eyes from AMD (age-related macular degeneration). Women who drink alcohol in moderate amounts are less likely to suffer from osteoporosis. Two antioxidants that are found in wine as well as in numerous plant foods, resveratrol and quercetin, slow down the growth of some cancer cells.

Of course, it probably is not that simple. The adverse effects of alcohol are obvious, and what is "moderate" to some is too little or too much to others. Wine drinkers tend to be more affluent than nondrinkers or heavy drinkers, and more likely to exercise and maintain a good diet. Thus, though there are real benefits to drinking wine, especially red wine, nondrinkers would probably be even better off by exercising and getting plenty of fruits and vegetables daily. All the phytonutrients that scientists have found in red wine are abundant in many fruits and vegetables. By adding a wide variety of these to your diet, as your Stone Age ancestors did, you'll have all the benefits that wine offers, at a lower cost and without the health risks of alcohol.

Sorting out the fiber factor

On a family trip to the zoo many years ago we happened to be at the gorilla habitat at feeding time. I was astonished at the huge mass of fruits and vegetables that was set before the lone ape in that particular enclosure. In the years since that visit I learned that Sam and Sal ate the equivalent amount of such food, although their selection was hardly as starchy as that modern ape's — or ours. Even more than their present-day equivalents, the fruits and vegetables of the past were very calorie-sparse, and Sam and Sal each needed from 3 to 5 pounds a day to fulfill their dietary needs. The fiber content of those primitive plant foods was greater than modern supermarket fare. The dietary differences between early humans and us are especially marked in terms of fiber. Their intake was about 10 times as high as that of contemporary Americans. Since that was what our bodies and theirs had evolved to utilize, the minuscule amount of fiber in our diet is bound to have biologic consequences.

Dr. Denis Burkitt, a South African physician, touted the benefits of a high-fiber diet more than half a century ago. He observed that in his own practice, spanning more than 40 years, he never saw a South African native on a typical native diet with appendicitis. When these same types of individuals moved to towns and cities and acquired urban lifestyles, they developed the ills of Westerners, including appendicitis.

In the 1940s, physicians noted that the rate of appendicitis decreased. It coincided with rationing, which forced people to eat less meat, and more high-fiber, protein- rich foods such as beans.

I noted the benefits of fiber in an earlier chapter. Except for that which senior citizens buy in boxes or bottles, fiber is accompanied by scores of phytonutrients, vitamins and minerals. Taken together, they form an important barrier against heart disease, which claims more than 1 million victims each year in the United States, and consumes an enormous share of our annual budget.

Fiber is related to lower risk of colon cancer but it's hard to sort out the reasons. For decades scientists assumed that fiber simply attached itself to cancer-causing substances in the bowel and kept them from contact with the intestinal lining. A study of more than 400,000 people attributed the 40 percent lower risk of colon cancer to fiber. Vitamins, antioxidants and other factors that are present in fiber-rich fruits and vegetables may also play a role. Salicylic acid, well known to everyone as aspirin, is present in fruits and vegetables, and vegetarians have a higher blood level of this chemical than nonvegetarians. The anti-inflammatory action of salicylic acid may help to prevent cancer of the colon and the pancreas. It could also help to explain why a high intake of fruits and vegetables reduces the risk of heart disease and stroke.

Puzzles among the pyramids

The Mediterranean Diet pyramid (Fig. 1, page 208) is less grain-based and more fruit- and vegetable-based than the USDA pyramid (Fig. 2, page 208). Note that beans, other legumes and nuts are in the second tier, and are not lumped together with animal meats. The prominence of this plant-based group is consistent with the Stone Age pyramid (Fig. 3, page 208), which has no grain group.

Red meat is at the top of the Mediterranean pyramid, which means that we should eat it sparingly. Meat was relatively scarce in the very early Stone Age, when early humans, not having tools of any kind, were mainly plant-eaters. Their sources of red meat in that era probably consisted mostly of carrion. When man became a toolmaker, his intake of red meat increased considerably. During the period in which we have placed Sam and Sal, about 50,000 years ago until the beginning of the agricultural age, humans became such efficient hunters that they eliminated some large game animals completely.

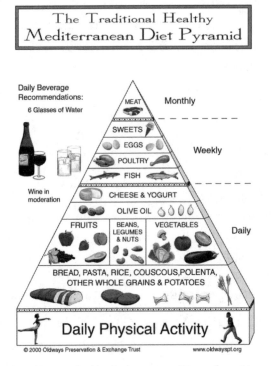

Figure 1: Mediterranean Diet pyramid

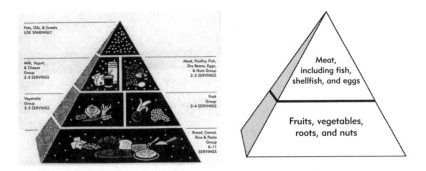

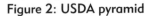

Figure 2: USDA pyramid   Figure 3: Stone Age pyramid

Sam and Sal didn't broil or fry their meat, but they may have been able to boil or steam their food. They probably roasted it over glowing coals, just like modern Americans do all summer long. That primitive practice may have some drawbacks, and not just because Dad's preference for almost-raw meat raises the risk of E. coli infection. That's an insignificant hazard compared to one associated with barbecuing: cancer of the intestine, breast, prostate, pancreas and liver.

When we brown, barbecue, broil or fry meat or other foods that contain creatinine and other substances in muscle, we cause the formation of chemicals called heterocyclic amines. These are powerful cancer-causing agents. Even though they are present in relatively small amounts, they may be additive to the role of fat in the formation of cancer cells. Frying at high temperatures for longer times produces high levels of heterocyclic amines, but barbecuing forms even greater amounts. There is a direct and strong correlation of the intake of well-done red meat with abnormalities of the colon (colorectal adenomas) that are precursors of colon cancer.

Confusing terms: creatine and creatinine

Creatine, *found in red meat, is a substance that is part of the energy-producing chemistry of muscle. Some athletes take it in the form of a supplement in order to improve short-term, high-intensity performance. There is no conclusive evidence that it is harmful in persons with normal kidneys.*

Creatinine *(note the extra syllable) is a by-product of creatine and accumulates in persons whose kidneys do not work properly.*

Among populations whose meat intake is low, the risk of colon cancer is also low. In Africa, where the intake of meat as a whole is less than 15 percent of that in the United States, the rate of colon cancer is approximately 10 percent of ours.

There is evidence that inhaling heterocyclic amines during the cooking process contributes to the high incidence of lung cancer among smokers.

Adding up the benefits of the Mediterranean diet

When we put all these factors together, the beneficial effects of the Mediterranean diet begin to come into focus. It's clear that persons who have a high intake of red meat and fat have an increased risk of various kinds of cancer and coronary artery disease. It's also an established fact that fruits and vegetables, with their high content of antioxidants, vitamins and other phytonutrients are protective against several types of malignancies. Their fiber content helps to lower cholesterol. The high levels of potassium in plant foods are associated with a lower risk of stroke. The cornucopia of antioxidants appears to lower cholesterol and the likelihood of a heart attack. Recent laboratory studies have shown that flavonoids found in citrus fruits, which are abundant in Mediterranean climates, have a specific inhibitory effect on the mutagenic (i.e., cancer-causing) activity of heterocyclic amines. Further, Mediterranean populations rely on olive oil for most of their added fat. Olive oil may contain a specific agent that inhibits the process by which cells become cancerous. The death rates from cancer of the prostate are low in those areas where consumption of olive oil is high.

To summarize, the diet of Crete and southern Italy is characterized by a low intake of red meat, and therefore provides relatively little exposure to factors that are associated with the development of cancer (heterocyclic amines) and heart disease (saturated fat). It contains a high level of fruits and vegetables, with their accompanying antioxidants and vitamins, some of which counteract the harmful effects of the toxic chemicals in meat. Vegetables, nuts and fish contain considerable amounts of omega-3 fatty acids, substances that protect against sudden cardiac death. Olive oil is rich in monosaturated fats and essential fatty acids, and may contain specific agents that protect against the development of cancer.

Thus, the Mediterranean area provides a dietary model that is consistent with the one on which Sam and Sal thrived. It is not just palatable but is enjoyable, and does not strain environmental resources. It is not the only healthful diet model, but its constituents are so familiar that it has been easy to hold it up as an example of what humans are meant to eat. Most Asian diets share the advantages of the Mediterranean, but Americans are less familiar with the foods of that vast area. The Japanese, whose good health and longevity are well known, use soy and salt heavily. The former is still almost a novelty for Westerners and the latter is associated with adverse health effects. Few in the United States are familiar with Middle Eastern foods, and even fewer have any knowledge concerning the staples of native Africans.

The diet pathway: what and how much

I have held up the Mediterranean diet as a model because it is convenient, well known and accepted by almost everyone, and inexpensive. If you follow the guidelines in Chapter Six, Supermarket Suicide and Restaurant Roulette, you will have adopted its major guidelines: lots of fruits and vegetables, some fish and lean meat, limited dairy products and only whole-grain baked goods. Save the sweets for le feste (feast days).

Stop thinking in terms of calories; think in fistfuls

Since even a registered dietician can't count calories exactly (Chapter Three), don't waste your time trying. Eat reasonable amounts and let your satiety mechanism take over. That's not as hard as it sounds.

A serving of meat or fish is about 4 ounces. That's about the size of my palm (not including fingers) in three dimensions. You probably are thinking that's not much help. Using that guideline, a hulking linebacker would probably eat about 4 times as much as a wispy gymnast. That's right, but don't you think that those proportions are just right for each of them? For these foods, if you limit your servings to those that are the size of your palm you won't overeat. Not even an average football player has a one-pound palm, but that's an average-sized steak in many restaurants.

Even the United States Department of Agriculture, which publishes *Dietary Guidelines for Americans* every 5 years, admits that "concepts like 30 percent of calories from fat are almost meaningless to the typical consumer." Don't eliminate all fat from your diet, but do eliminate grossly fatty foods. That includes fried food and bacon. Find substitutes for butter, margarine and mayonnaise. Whether eating at home or dining out, choose lean cuts of meat and trim away the obvious fat in other kinds.

For fruits and vegetables, think of fist-sized servings. An apple is about the size of an average person's clenched fist, which I call a fistful just for illustration. So is a banana. (Use your imagination.) If you're big enough to be a tackle for the Dallas Cowboys, it probably takes 2 bananas to make a fistful. That's appropriate for your body mass, and you won't overdo it if you always eat 2 bananas instead of 1. You can apply this rule to potatoes, broccoli, corn or beans, or any other cooked vegetable.

Leafy salads (not the kind you serve with a spoon) entitle you to 2 fistfuls, because they are calorie-sparse and contain lots of phytonutrients and fiber. Spoon-type salads are usually high in fat, which is what holds them together. If you insist, eat them sparingly.

Nutritionists urge us to have 9 servings a day of fruits and vegetables. Nine fistfuls is a generous amount. That's lots of stomach-filling fiber and will keep you from feeling hungry between meals.

A fistful of pizza dough should yield the base for about three average slices and about 750 calories.

If you gently ball up 2 slices of bread the volume will be about the size of an average fist. That's 2 servings, according to the USDA Food Guide Pyramid.

The fist of a 160-pound person has a volume of about 12 ounces. That much milk will give you about 450 milligrams of calcium, or about one-third of most persons' daily needs. A 12-ounce can of soda will give you no calcium and about 140 empty calories.

Five fistfuls of water (60 ounces) will meet the needs of the average-sized person on an average spring day doing aver-

> Determine the volume of your own fist. Place your clenched fist into a large measuring pitcher and add water to the 20-ounce mark. Remove your hand and note the volume of water that remains. The difference is the volume of your fist and will probably be about 12 ounces.

age activity. For bigger bodies, hotter days and more activity use the urine-quality rule that I described earlier: if your urine has a strong odor or color, you need more fluids. It should be light yellow or straw-colored, with little odor.

Eat slowly, just as your mother told you to. Each of us has a satiety mechanism that quenches our appetite, but it takes about 20 minutes to take effect. People who eat slowly do eat less, and they are not likely to be hungry enough for an enormous dessert.

If you really think you need to lose weight

This book does not include a detailed weight-loss program. *Health Secrets of the Stone Age* gives an explanation of how our bodies have evolved within the environment that nature has provided, and how we can maintain that relationship in spite of modern changes in that environment. Given that most of us are overweight, some of us are obese, and all of us want to look better and feel better, I offer some specific guidelines for the person who is interested in losing weight, or more precisely, fat.

Pick a reasonable, attainable, safe target for total weight loss

Plan on taking off no more than 10 percent of your present weight in the first phase. When you have reached that goal you can set another one. Aim for a weight loss of about 2 pounds per week in order to avoid fatigue, cravings and other diet discomforts.

Two pounds per week doesn't sound like much, but that's 25 pounds in only 3 months, a significant drop for a 250-pounder. Based on my experience with seminar audiences, most people would be happy to lose about 10 pounds. That may seem modest, but it's associated with a considerable lowering of risk of heart disease and diabetes.

Eat between meals

In the absence of vigorous exercise, taking in one to three large meals a day raises the level of blood sugar that in turn raises levels of insulin. Insulin promotes fat storage and has several other effects that over several years result in diabetes and heart disease. In only 2 simple steps you can keep blood sugar and insulin levels low and keep your energy level high. First, discard the old idea of simple versus complex carbohydrates. That's an outmoded concept. Shop mainly for low-GI (Glycemic Index) foods, which I described in Chapter Five and listed in Appendix 3. When you learn how to find them in the grocery store you'll know how to locate them on the menu. Second, keep plenty of snack foods around (see sidebar, p. 215). Between-meal cravings are the undoing of dieters. Easy access to satisfying, healthy snacks helps to avoid distracting hunger pangs.

There may be an explanation for those uncomfortable sensations. When the stomach is empty it produces a hormone called ghrelin. Blood levels of this hormone rise during hunger and fall after a meal. Long-term food restriction causes elevated ghrelin levels that may drive the appetite, intensify cravings, and make it impossible for most persons to keep weight off. If frequent snacking inhibits the rise in ghrelin it might explain why persons who nibble instead of gorge are less likely to regain the weight they have lost.

Sensible snacks — keep 'em handy

- *Keep fruit on hand at all times. That includes your workplace. Apples stay fairly fresh for weeks.*
- *Make snack foods attractive and inviting. My wife keeps 3 small glass containers on the coffee table in the family room. One contains walnuts, the second holds almonds and the third, dried fruit. The nuts are rich in omega-3 fatty acids, and the dried fruit is rich in fiber. (N.B.: Some dried fruit is also high in calories. A single fig has about 45, one prune has about 20, a date has about 8 and an apricot half about 4.)*
- *Protein bars travel well and keep for a long time. One bar can provide 2 snacks a day, each with about 10 grams of protein and little or no fat. Pick the ones with low carbohydrate.*
- *Although baby carrots have a relatively high Glycemic Index, a small handful will not give you a sugar high. Even a medium-sized adult carrot has only about 30 calories. That's less than 2 Hershey's chocolate kisses. Carrots also have lots of vitamin A and C and other antioxidants.*
- *A teaspoon of peanut butter has only about 30 calories. Put it on celery to give it a nicer texture.*
- *Natural, unsweetened applesauce generously piled onto a slice of angel food cake is a nice accompaniment to a cup of tea.*
- *Nonfat cottage cheese with pineapple, strawberries, blueberries or other fruit provides a tasty source of calcium.*
- *A whole-grain bagel with a slice of turkey will stave off cravings longer than some other snacks, but use mustard instead of mayonnaise if it needs a little extra flavor, and add a slice of tomato.*
- *Plain popcorn is a safe snack, except for the packaged forms that contain butter, cheese and salt.*

Make most of your snacks high in protein, with almost no fat and little carbohydrate

Protein will not only keep you from losing mass from your muscles and other important organs, it will help you to avoid the fatigue that dieters usually experience. Most dieters make the mistake of cutting back on all three macronutrients (fat, protein, carbohydrate), but your need for protein doesn't go down when you fast. You still need it to replace cells that wear out and to make antibodies that fight infection. When your protein intake remains the same, as your carbohydrate and fat intake go down, you are not on a high protein diet. As you cut back significantly on caloric intake, percentages become meaningless, and absolute numbers matter most.

Protein: how much do you really need?

The average person requires a minimum of 20 to 30 grams of protein daily. For an active, 150-pound person, the optimal amount of protein is about 50 to 100 grams (0.3 to 0.6 grams of protein per pound of body weight). Those who exercise regularly require the higher amount. A palm-sized portion (4 ounces) of fish contains a little more than 20 grams; a similar portion of chicken contains about 30. Four ounces of eye round beef contain about 32 grams; 1 cup of kidney beans contains about 15; a whole egg contains about 6. Most protein bars contain about 20 grams.

All protein is not the same. Most animal protein sources contain all the essential amino acids, but some vegetables (such as corn) do not. Vegetarians should be certain that their diet contains a large assortment of protein-containing foods. Sam and Sal had a wide selection of animals (including insects) and vegetables from which to choose. Protein deficiency among preagricultural peoples was rare. That remains true of hunter-gatherers today.

Most healthy persons tolerate a high-protein diet well, but there is no point in taking in more than you need. A high-protein diet may be associated with loss of calcium, and it is definitely detrimental to those with liver or kidney disease.

Protein food bars are an excellent choice. They are convenient to store and carry and come in a wide variety of flavors.

Unfortunately, many of them are so unpalatable that some people give up on them.

Don't think of exercise, think of movement

Sam and Sal were in motion almost continually. Our bodies did not evolve toward a state of immobility, and we must recognize that there is an exquisite interaction between movement and optimal health. The consequences of inactivity are enormous.

I favor a program of daily exercise, alternating between walking and resistance exercises, not because I think it's what our ancestors did, but because it fulfills our bodily requirements without disrupting our lifestyle. For those who cannot take the time for an organized regimen, Minirobics™ provide a partial solution.

A pedometer helps to measure activity. If you know how many steps you take in a day it's easier to find ways of increasing that number. Give yourself a target above your baseline and strive to increase it every week. Remember that walking is the primary form of activity in some hunter-gatherer groups. Action doesn't have to be extreme in order to be fruitful. Burning only a hundred extra calories a day will help you to take off almost a pound every month. You can accomplish that in 30 or 40 minutes, and you don't even have to do it in one session.

Have a strategy for avoiding high-fat, high-sugar foods

They do not trigger your satiety mechanism. In other words, when you eat sweet and/or fatty foods you don't start to feel full until you've had more than your body requires. The guidelines for lowering fat intake that I gave in Chapter Six are not just theoretically sound, they work. However, they won't work without commitment. That's why it's important for anyone who wants to lose weight to set a realistic goal, write it down, and post it where he or she can see it every day.

Have some ready-made strategies. When I find myself in a fast-food restaurant (it happens) I ask them to hold the fries. Hunger and temptation are a terrible combination.

Make dessert a once-a-week treat, and try to make that only fruit.

Keep your dieting strategy to yourself and share it only with your family

You'll need their cooperation and understanding. Since being overweight often involves more than one family member it might be easier than you think to get their help. On the other hand, broadcasting to others that you're on a diet brings out the Martyr Mentality (Chapter Three).

Maintain the proper mindset

Remind yourself that carrying excess weight for most of a person's lifetime is a relatively recent phenomenon in evolutionary terms. Although it has many causes it is entirely preventable, as hunter-gatherer (i.e., Stone Age) humans demonstrate.

Stifle stress

The people like Sam and Sal who lived 50,000 years ago encountered some stress in their lives, but it was orders of magnitude less than that which we encounter now. They had access to an abundance of wild game and plant foods. They weren't concerned about starving to death. Population pressure and crowding did not exist, as most humans of that epoch existed in small bands of less than 40 or 50 persons.

That is not to say that there was no stress. Fossils records clearly show that many of Sam and Sal's contemporaries died of injury caused by other humans. Certainly some of them must have perished as another animal's meal, but those carnivores didn't leave many clues behind. It was just these kinds of sudden terrors that determined the fight or flight adaptation that involves so many bodily responses. But they were occasional threats, not sustained ones. In between, they led lives like those of modern hunter-gatherers who still live in small bands. The rise in blood pressure, the quickened pulse and the adrenalin surge that occurred as they chased down an antelope or a bison subsided by the time they had carried the still-warm carcass back to that day's campsite. They didn't have to hunt, or even to gather, every single day, just as modern African bushmen or Australian aborigines do not. And when darkness came, they nestled together protectively, shared the day's experiences, and slept until they were rested.

An alarm clock wakens today's office-bound hunter before daylight and the adrenalin surge continues beyond sunset. The stress lasts every working day. Those who cross time zones and who work night shifts disrupt the biologic rhythm that has taken hundreds of thousands of years to evolve.

Westerners ignore these changes but they clearly contribute to the stress-related diseases that involve the heart and the immune system. Several hormones such as growth hormone and testosterone fluctuate hourly according to a blueprint that evolved well over a million years ago. There are daily and seasonal hormonal patterns that are based on cycles of light and darkness. During the hundreds of thousands of years during which our body systems developed, our only light source was the sun. This day-night pattern determined our body rhythm, known as the *circadian* rhythm. Anyone who has experienced the discomfort of jet lag can appreciate what happens when we reverse the normal sequence of activity and sleep. Electric lighting is adequate for most visual performance, but it's not appropriate for a normal sleep/wake cycle.

Shift work is inescapable for some persons, especially those who provide emergency services such as police and fire protection, and medical services. We will never be able to eliminate the need for work schedules that are contrary to the body's natural sleep cycles, but there is clearly a need to reduce the effects of such a lifestyle. Short-term symptoms are similar to those of jet lag: disturbed sleep, daytime drowsiness, diminished alertness, and intestinal disturbances.

Long-term problems include a higher incidence of heart disease among persons who work at night and sleep by day. Night shift work and exposure to light increase the production of estrogen. This may be the reason why women who work at night and have more exposure to artificial light have a higher rate of breast cancer than those who do not.

Shift workers must eat during the hours when they are on duty, but the way that our bodies utilize food that is eaten at night is different from that of daytime meals. Production of vital hormones such as insulin, thyroid hormone, cortisol and several other hormones differs with respect to time of day. This may explain why type 2 diabetes and hypertension occur earlier, and are more severe, in persons who undergo long periods with inadequate sleep, and why shift workers have a higher incidence of heart disease.

It isn't necessary to remind today's audience that stress is part of modern life and that it contributes to various illnesses. Popular authors such as Dr. Dean Ornish and Dr. Andrew Weil emphasize that loving relationships and stress reduction influence both the incidence and outcome of diseases that include infection, immune disorders, heart disease and cancer. Medical scientists are delving into these issues at an unprecedented rate. The United States Library of Medicine lists over one-half million entries under the topic of stress. It's comforting to know that relieving stress is not complicated or expensive, and we can learn a great deal from ancient as well as contemporary models.

In the wonderful book by Frances Mayes, *Under the Tuscan Sun*, a meal does not simply provide nourishment, it is a celebration. It is often an excuse to gather with friends and family over a prolonged midday or evening feast. Preparing the food may take hours, perhaps a day or two, but what does it matter, especially if it involves the camaraderie of kitchen companions? What a contrast with drive-through fast food, microwave meals and delivered pizza. When Sam and Sal ate, perhaps several times a day, there was no reason to hurry. Now we face schedules, deadlines and days filled with conferences. We eat at our desks, or even in the car. Few employees have the luxury of unlimited time for workday meals.

Americans who visit Latin countries view the siesta as an annoyance. Most banks, businesses and tourist attractions close for about two hours. Unfortunately, competition for the United States dollar has eliminated the siesta in many cities. Almost no one recognizes the fact that the siesta developed as an evolutionary survival mechanism. When we are active in the hours that follow a meal we use up calories that we would otherwise store up either as glycogen or as fat deposits. The glycogen is available as short-term energy, and the fat as long-term energy. When we rest after a meal we replenish them. Sam and Sal didn't eat beyond satiety, so their accumulation of stored energy was not excessive even if they enjoyed a siesta every day.

Persons who travel outside the United States sometimes comment on or complain about the slower pace in other countries. Meetings that don't begin on time, stores whose hours are inconsistent with the posted schedule, business conferences in which small talk precedes serious discussion all seem to reflect a lackadaisical attitude. That is consistent with an ancient lifestyle that was devoid of deadlines and free from chronic stress — the Stone Age lifestyle.

The pathway to health that I described in this chapter seems deceptively simple to an audience that is used to entire books on diet manipulation, counting calories, avoidance of certain food combinations and selecting foods according to blood type. The overworked expression "this is not rocket science" perfectly describes my attitude toward health maintenance. We may not know all the reasons why lifestyles from the Mediterranean Sea to the mountains of Okinawa result in a long life span and few chronic diseases, but we only have to imitate some of their features in order to enjoy their benefits. We don't need a Ph.D. in muscle physiology to recognize that persons who exercise are healthier and happier than those who do not. Nor do we have to measure every choice with "Could I eat this if I were naked with a sharp stick on the savanna?" as proposed by one author, not entirely tongue-in-cheek. Instead, take a pleasant walk with a dear companion, use a little sharp stick to spear another olive, and enjoy a glass of Chianti.

References

Chapter One

Braunwald E et al., Eds., *Harrison's Principles of Internal Medicine*, 15th ed., McGraw Hill, 2000

Eaton SB et al., "Evolutionary Health Promotion," *Preventive Medicine* 2002; 34:109–118

Peery TM, "The New and Old Diseases: A Study of Mortality Trends in the United States, 1900–1969," *Am J Clin Path* 1975 April; 63:453–74

White PD, "Coronary Heart Disease: Then and Now," *JAMA* 1969 Feb 26; 203:9:282–83

Kochanek KD et al., "Deaths: Preliminary Data for 1999," *National Vital Statistics Reports* 2001 June; 49(3): 1–5

Cohen MN and Armelagos GJ, Eds., *Paleopathology at the Origins of Agriculture*, Academic Press 1984

Diamond J, *The Third Chimpanzee*, Harper Perennial, publ., 1993

Cordain L, "Cereal Grains: Humanity's Double-Edged Sword, in Evolutionary Aspects of Nutrition and Health, Diet, Exercise, Genetics and Chronic Disease," *World Rev Nutr Diet*, Simopoulos AP, Ed., Karger publ., Basel 1999 vol. 84:19–73

Cordain L, "Scant evidence of periodic starvation among hunter-gatherers," *Diabetologia* 1999; 42:383–4

Smith U, "Life style and genes — the key factors for diabetes and the metabolic syndrome," *J Int Med* 1992;232:99–01

Strong JP et al., "Pathological Determinants of Atherosclerosis in Youth Research Group, Natural History of Aortic and Coronary Atherosclerotic Lesions in Youth," *Arteriosclerosis and Thrombosis* 1993 Sept 113; 9:1291–98

Eaton SB, Konner M and Shostak M, "Stone Agers in the fast lane: chronic degenerative diseases in evolutionary perspective," *Amer J Med* 1988 April; 84:739–49

Trowell HC and Burkitt DP, *Western diseases: their emergence and prevention*, Harvard Univ. Press, 1981

Rode A and Shephard RJ, "Modernization of lifestyle, body fat content and body fat distribution: a comparison of Igloolik Inuit and Volochanka nGanasan," *Int. J. Obes Relat Metab Disord* 1995 Oct;19(10): 709–16

West KM, "Diabetes in American Indians and Other Native Populations of the New World," *Diabetes* 1974 Oct; 23:10:841–55

McDougall JA, *The McDougall Program*, Penguin Books, New York, 1990

Tominaga S and Kuroishi T, "Epidemiology of breast cancer in Japan," *Cancer Letters* 1995; 90(1):75–79

Kohrle J et al., "Selenium in Biology: Facts and Medical Perspectives," *Biol Chem.* 2000 September/October, 381:849–864

Harlan JR, "A wild wheat harvest in Turkey," *Archeology*, 1967, 197–201

Diamond J, *Guns, Germs and Steel*, Norton publ., New York, 1999

Reuters, "Biodiversity Shrinks as Farm Breeds Die Out," 2001 Sept 22

The Doctor's Book of Food Remedies, Yeager S Ed., p. 334–5, Rodale Press 1998

"Acceleration in obesity," *Nutrition Action* Jan/Feb 2001

Beil L, "Girth of a Nation," *Dallas Morning News* 1999 Aug 29

Press release, "Sugar intake hit all-time high in 1999," Center for Science in the Public Interest, 2000 May 18

Pennington JA, *Bowes and Church's Food Values of Portions Commonly Used*, 1998, 17th ed., Lippincott, New York

Eaton SB et al., "Stone Agers in the Fast Lane: Chronic Degenerative Diseases in Evolutionary Perspective," *Amer J Med* April 1988; 84:739–49

Tannahill R, *Food in History*, Three Rivers Press 1988, p. 23

O'Keefe JH and Cordain L, "Cardiovascular Disease Resulting from a Diet and Lifestyle at Odds with Our Paleolithic Genome: How to Become a 21st-Century Hunter-Gatherer," *Mayo Clin Proc* 2004; 79:101–108

Roosevelt AC, "Population, Health and the Evolution of Subsistence" in Cohen MN and Armelagos GJ, Eds., *Paleopathology at the Origins of Agriculture*, p. 586, Academic Press 1984

Bennett PH, "Type 2 diabetes among the Pima Indians of Arizona: An epidemic attributable to environmental change?" *Nutr Rev* 1999; 57:5:S51–S54

Valencia ME et al., "The Pima Indians in Sonora, Mexico," *Nutr Rev* 1999; 57(5): S55–S58

Chapter Two

Miller GJ, "Postprandial lipaemia and haemostatic factors," *Arteriosclerosis* 1998 Dec; 141 Suppl 1: S47–51

Hozumi T et al., "Change in Coronary Flow Reserve on Transthoracic Doppler Echocardiography after a Single High-Fat Meal in Young Healthy Men," *Ann Int Med* 2002 April; 136(7):523–528

Kennedy ET et al., "Popular diets: Correlation to health, nutrition and obesity," *J Am Diet Assoc* 2001; 101:411–420

Greenwood CE, "Cognitive impairment in rats fed high fat diets: A specific effect of saturated fatty acid intake," *Behav Neurosci* 1996; 110:451–59

Sinaki M and Lynn SG, "Reducing the risk of falls through proprioceptive dynamic posture training in osteoporotic women with kyphotic posturing," *Am J Phys Med Rehab* 2002; 81(4): 241–46

Guyton AC and Hall JE, *Textbook of Medical Physiology*, Tenth Ed., 2000, WB Saunders publ.

Evans W and Rosenberg IH, *Biomarkers*, 1992, Simon and Schuster publ.

Sher L, "Exercise, well-being and endogenous molecules of mood," *Lancet* 1996 Aug 17; 348:477

Blake AJ et al., "Accuracy of food portion estimation by overweight and normal-weight subjects," *J Am Dietetic Assoc* 1989 Jul; 89(7): 962–4

Cooper RK and Cooper LL, *Low-Fat Living*, Rodale Press, 1996, p. 26)

Chapter Three

Cordain L et al., "Scant evidence of periodic starvation among hunter-gatherers," *Diabetologia* 1999; 42:383–384

Uauy R, Albala C and Kain J, "Obesity trends in Latin America: transiting from under- to overweight," *J Nutr* 2001 Mar; 131(3): 893S–899S

Pavlou KN et al., "Physical activity as a supplement to a weight-loss dietary regimen," *Am J Clin Nutr* 1989; 49:1110–14

Brugman E et al., "Dieting, weight and health in adolescents in the Netherlands," *Int J Obesity* 1997; 21:54–60

Guyton AC and Hall JE, *Textbook of Medical Physiology*, 2001, p. 809, W. Saunders publ., New York

Petersmarck KA et al., "The effect of weight cycling on blood lipids and blood pressure in the Multiple Risk Factor Intervention Special Intervention Group," *Int J Obes Relat Metab Disord* 1999 Dec; 23(12): 1246–1255

Guagnano MT et al., "Risk factors for hypertension in obese women. The role of weight cycling," *Eur J Clin Nutr* 2000 Apr; 54(4): 356–360

Blackburn GL and Borrazzo ECL, "Weight Cycling," *J Amer Med Assoc* 1995 April 5; 273(13): 998

Mokdad AH et al., "The Continuing Epidemic of Obesity in the United States," *J Amer Med Assoc* 284:13:1519, Oct. 4, 2000

Jain A et al., "Why don't low-income mothers worry about their preschoolers being overweight?" *Pediatrics* 2001 May 107:5: 1138–1146

Kennedy ET et al., "Popular diets: correlation to health, nutrition and obesity," *J Am Diet Assoc* 2001 Apr; 101(4): 411–20

Schlundt DG et al., "The role of breakfast in the treatment of obesity," *Am J Clin Nutr* 1992; 55:645–51

Murphy JM et al., "The relationship of school breakfast to psychosocial and academic functioning," *Arch Pediatr Adolesc Med* 152:899–907, 1998

Pasman WJ et al., "Effect of two breakfasts, different in carbohydrate composition, on hunger and satiety and mood in healthy men," *Int J Obes Relat Metabol Disord* 2003 Jun; 27(6):663–8

Pollitt E et al., "Fasting and Cognitive Function," *J Psychiatr Res* 1982; 17(2): 169–174

Wolever S et al., "Second-meal effect: low glycemic index foods eaten at dinner improve subsequent breakfast glycemic response," *Am J Clin Nut* 48:1041–1047, 1988

Black AE and Cole TJ, "Biased over- or under-reporting is characteristic of individuals whether over time or by different assessment methods," *J Am Diet Assoc* 2001;101:70–80

Blake AJ et al., "Accuracy of food portion estimation by over-weight and normal-weight subjects," *J Am Diet Assoc* 1989 Jul; 89(7): 962–4

Mertz W et al., "What are people really eating? The relation between energy intake derived from estimated diet record intake determined to maintain body weight," *Am J Clin Nut* 1991 Aug; 54(2): 291–295

Pennington JA, *Food Values of Portions Commonly Used*, 17th ed. 1998, Lippincott Williams and Wilkins

Kobayashi H et al., "Visceral fat accumulation contributes to insulin resistance, small-sized low-density lipoprotein, and pro-gression of coronary artery disease in middle-aged non-obese Japanese men," *Jpn Circ J* 2001 Mar; 65(3): 193–9

Popkin BM and Doak CM, "The Obesity Epidemic Is a World-wide Phenomenon," *Nutr Rev* 1998 Apr; 56(4): 106–114

Mokdad AH et al., "The Spread of the Obesity Epidemic in the United States, 1991–1998," *J Amer Med Assoc* Oct. 27, 1999: 282 (16) 1519–1522

Schelkin PH, "The Risks of Riding the Weight Loss Rollercoaster," *The Physician and Sportsmedicine* 1991 Jun; 19:6:154

Brownell KD and Rodin J, "Medical, metabolic and psychological effects of weight cycling," *Arch Intern Med* 1994 June 27; 154(12): 1325–1330

Syngal S et al., "Long-term weight patterns and risk for cholecystectomy in women," *Ann Intern Med* 1999 Mar 16; 130(6): 471–7

Greenberger NJ and Paumgartner G in *Harrison's Principles of Internal Medicine*, 15th ed., p. 1777, 2001

Erlinger S, "Gallstones in obesity and weight loss," *Eur J Gastro-enterol Hepatol* 2000 Dec; 12(12): 1347–52

Wurtman RJ and Wurtman JJ, "Brain Serotonin, Carbohydrate-craving, Obesity and Depression," *Adv Exp Med Biol* 1996; 398:35–41

Mattes RD and Bormann LA, "Reduced dietary underrecording with concurrent tracking of hunger," *J Amer Dietetic Assoc* 101 (5); 578–9, May 2001

Anderson JW et al., "Health advantages and disadvantages of weight-reducing diets: a computer analysis and critical review," *J Am Coll Nutr* 2000 Oct; 19(5): 578–90

Reddy ST et al., "Effect of Low-Carbohydrate High-Protein Diets on Acid-Base Balance, Stone-Forming Propensity, and Calcium Metabolism," *Am J Kidney Dis* 2002 Aug; 40(2): 265–74

Kwiterovich PO et al., "Effect of a High-Fat Ketogenic Diet on Plasma Levels of Lipids, Lipoproteins, and Apolipoproteins in Children," *J Am Med Assoc* 2003 Aug 20;290(7):912–920

Best TH et al., "Cardiac complications in pediatric patients on the ketogenic diet," *Neurology* 2000 Jun; 54(12):2328–30

Landers P et al., "Effect of weight loss plans on body composition and diet duration," *J Okla State Med Assoc* 2002 May; 95(5): 329–31

Benton D and Nabb S, "Carbohydrate, Memory and Mood," *Nutr Rev* 2003 May; 61(5):S61–S67

"Heart Association to warn against low-carb diets," CNN.com web posting, March 20, 2001

Blaak E, "Gender differences in fat metabolism," *Curr Opin Clin Nutr Metab Care* 2001 Nov; 4(6): 499–502

Tattersall I and Matternes JH, "Once we were not alone," *Scientific American* 2000 January; 56–62

Chapter Four

Balady GJ, "Survival of the Fittest — More Evidence," 2002 Mar 14, *N Engl J Med* 346(11): 852–3

Scott WA and Couzens GS, "Treating Injuries in Active Seniors," *Phys/Sports* 1996 May; 24:5:63–68

Bales CW and Ritchie CS, "Sarcopenia, Weight Loss, and Nutritional Frailty in the Elderly," *Annu Rev Nutr* 2002; 22:309–23

Vincent KR et al., "Resistance Exercise and Physical Performance in Adults Aged 60 to 83," *J Am Geriatr Soc* 2002; 50:1100–1107

Booth FW et al., "Waging war on physical inactivity: using modern molecular ammunition against an ancient enemy," *J Appl Physiol* 2002; 93:3–20

Serdula MK et al., "The Association between Fruit and Vegetable Intake and Chronic Disease Risk Factors," *Epidemiology* 1996; 7:161–165

Roubenoff R and Castaneda C, "Sarcopenia – Understanding the Dynamics of Aging Muscle," *J Am Med Assoc* 2001 Sept 12; 286(10): 1230–1231

Work JA, "Strength Training: A Bridge to Independence for the Elderly," *The Physician and Sportsmedicine* 1989 Nov; 17(11): 134–40

Evans W and Rosenberg IH, *Biomarkers*, Simon and Schuster publ., 1992

Janssen I et al., "Low relative skeletal muscle mass (sarcopenia) in older persons is associated with functional impairment and physical disability," *J Amer Geriatr Soc* 2002 May; 50(5): 889–96

Hurley BF and Roth SM, "Strength training in the elderly; effects on risk factors for age-related diseases," *Sports Med* 2000 October; 30(4) 249–268

Beniamini Y et al., "High-intensity strength training of patients enrolled in an outpatient cardiac rehabilitation program," *J Cardiopulmon Rehabil* 1999 Jan; 19(1): 8–17

Eaton SB et al., "Paleolithic Nutrition," *N Engl J Med* 1985; 312:5:283–89

Stewart KS, "Exercise Training and the Cardiovascular Consequences of Type 2 Diabetes and Hypertension," *J Am Med Assoc* 2002 Oct 2; 288(13): 1622–31

Colberg SR et al., "Chronic exercise is associated with enhanced cutaneous blood flow in type 2 diabetes," *J Diabetes Complications* 2002 Mar–Apr; 16(2): 139–45

Meyer TJ, "Evaluation and Management of Insomnia," *Hospital Practice* 1998 December 15; 33(12): 75–86

Singh NA et al., "A Randomized Controlled Trial on the Effect of Exercise on Sleep," *Sleep* 1997; 20(2): 95–101

Slemenda C et al., "Quadriceps weakness and osteoarthritis of the knee," *Ann Int Med* 1997 Jul 15; 127(2): 97–104

Avunduk A et al., "The Comparisons of Intraocular Pressure Reductions after Isometric and Isokinetic Exercises in Normal Individuals," *Ophthalmologica* 1999; 213: 290–294

Evans WJ, "Exercise-induced skeletal muscle damage," *The Physician and Sportsmedicine*, 15:1: 89–100, Jan 87

Barlas P et al., "Managing delayed-onset muscle soreness: lack of effect of selected oral systemic analgesics," *Arch Phys Med Rehabil* 81(7) 966–72, July 2000

Thompson D et al., "Prolonged vitamin C supplementation and recovery from demanding exercise," *Int J Sport Nutr Exerc Metab* 2001 Dec; 11(4): 466–81

Pavlou K, "Exercise as an adjunct to weight loss and maintenance in moderately obese subjects," *Am. J. Clin. Nut.* 1989; 49:1115–1123

Link MS et al., "Ventricular arrhythmias in the athlete," *Curr Opin Cardiol* 2001 Jan; 16(1): 30–39

Gunnarson OT and Judge JO, "Exercise at midlife: How and why to prescribe it for sedentary patients," *Geriatrics* 1997 May; 52(5): 71–80

Manson JE et al., "Walking Compared with Vigorous Exercise for the Prevention of Cardiovascular Events in Women," *N Eng J Med* 2002 Sep 5; 347(10): 716–25

Hurley BF and Roth SM, "Strength Training in the Elderly," *Sports Med* 2000; 30(4): 249–268

Lambert D, *The Field Guide to Early Man*, Diagram Group, publ., 2002

Das UN, "The Brain-Lipid-Heart Connection," *Nutrition* 2001; 17(3) 260–262

Grieve JS and Ko WM, "Energy expenditure during walking and jogging," *J Sports Med Phys Fitness* 2000 Dec; 40(4): 297–302

Cooper R, *Low-Fat Living*, 1996, Rodale Press publ., p. 49

Kemmler W et al., "Benefits of 2 Years of Intense Exercise on Bone Density, Physical Fitness, and Blood Lipids in Early Post-menopausal Osteopenic Women," *Arch Int Med* 2004 May 24; 164:1084–1091

Nelson ME et al., "Effects of High-Intensity Strength Training on Multiple Risk Factors for Osteoporotic Fractures," *J Am Med Assoc* 1994 Dec 28; 272(24): 1909–1914

Sinaki M et al., "Stronger back muscles reduce the incidence of vertebral fractures: a prospective 10-year follow-up of post-menopausal women," *Bone* 2002 Jun; 30(6):836–41

Boulé NG et al., "Effects of Exercise on Glycemic Control and Body Mass in Type 2 Diabetes Mellitus: A Meta-analysis of Controlled Clinical Trials," *J Am Med Assoc* 2001 Sept 12; 286(10): 1218–1227

Eaton SB and Eaton SB III, "Paleolithic vs. modern diets — selected pathophysiological implications," *Eur J Nutr* 2000; 39: 67070

Nelson ME et al., "Effects of high-intensity strength training on multiple risk factors for osteoporotic fractures," *J Am Med Assoc*, 1994 Dec 28; 272(24) 1909–14

Youngstedt SD et al., "Is sleep disturbed by vigorous late-night exercise?" *Med Sci Sports Exerc* 1999 June; 31(6): 864–869

King AC et al., "Moderate-intensity exercise and self-rated quality of sleep in older adults," *J Am Med Assoc* 1997; 277(1): 32–37

Washington RL et al., "Strength Training by Children and Adolescents," *Pediatrics* 2001 June 6; 107(6): 1470–72

Matthews CE et al., "Moderate to vigorous physical activity and risk of upper-respiratory tract infection," *Med Sci Sports Exerc* 2002 Aug; 34(8): 1242–48

Chapter Five

Powers AC, "Diabetes Mellitus," in Braunwald E et al., *Harrison's Principles of Internal Medicine*, 15th ed., McGraw Hill publ., 2000, p. 2114

Rosenbloom A et al., (Consensus Panel), "Type 2 Diabetes in Children and Adolescents," *Pediatrics* 2000 Mar; 105(3): 671–80

Wild S et al., "Global Prevalence of Diabetes," *Diabetes Care* 2004 May; 27(5):1047–1053

Rosenbloom AL et al., "Emerging epidemic of type 2 diabetes in youth," *Diabetes Care* 1999 Feb; 22(2): 345–54

Goran MJ, "Metabolic precursors and effects of obesity in children: a decade of progress, 1990–1999," *Am J Clin Nutr* 2001; 73:158–71

Kochanek KS et al., "Deaths: Preliminary Data for 1999," *National Vital Statistics Reports*, 49:3, June 26, 2001

Brosnan CA et al., "Type 2 Diabetes in Children and Adolescents: An Emerging Disease," *J Pediatr Health Care* 2001 Jul-Aug; 15(4): 187–93

American Diabetes Association Panel, "Type 2 Diabetes in Children and Adolescents," *Pediatrics* 2000, 105:3; 671–680

Bruce WR et al., "Possible mechanisms relating diet and the risk of colon cancer," *Cancer Epidemiol Biomarkers Prep*, 2000, 9(12): 1271–9

McCarty MF, "Insulin secretion as a determinant of pancreatic cancer risk," *Med Hypotheses* 2001; 57(2): 146–50

Rhoades ER, "Changing Paradigms and Their Effect on American Indian and Alaska Native Health," *Ann Epidemiol* 1997; 7:227–229

Shell ER, "The New World Syndrome," *The Atlantic Monthly*, p. 50–53, June 2001

West KM, "Diabetes in American Indians and Other Native Populations of the New World," *Diabetes* 1974; 23; 10:841–855

Bell RA, "An Epidemiologic Review of Dietary Intake Studies among American Indians and Alaska Natives; Implications for Heart Disease and Cancer Risk," *Ann Epidemiol*, 1997; 7; 4:229–240

Bennett PH, "Type 2 Diabetes among the Pima Indians of Arizona: An Epidemic Attributable to Environmental Change?" *Nutr Rev* 1999; 57(5) S51–S54

Rode A and Shephard RJ, "Modernization of lifestyle, body fat content and body fat distribution: a comparison of Igloolik Inuit and Volochanka nGanasan," *Int J Obes Relat Metab Disord* 1995; 19(10): 709–16

Valencia ME et al., "The Pima Indians in Sonora, Mexico," *Nutrition Reviews* 1999; 57:5:S55–S58

Esparza J et al., "Daily Energy Expenditure in Mexican and USA Pima Indians: low physical activity as a possible cause of obesity," *Internet J Obesity* 2000; 24:55–59

Nishikawa T et al., "The missing link: a single unifying mechanism for diabetic complications," *Kidney Int* 2000 Sep; 58 Suppl 77: S26–30

Gugliucci A, "Glycation as the glucose link to diabetic complications," *J Am Osteopath Assoc* 2000 Oct; 100(10): 621–34

Swanson JE et al., "Metabolic effects of dietary fructose in healthy subjects," *Am J Clin Nutr* 1992; 55:851–6

Hallfrisch J, "Fructose and blood cholesterol," *Am J Clin Nutr*, 1993; 57(1): 89

Rendell M, "Dietary Treatment of Diabetes Mellitus" (editorial), *New Engl J Med* 2000, 342:19; 1440–41

Benini L et al., "Gastric emptying of a solid meal is accelerated by the removal of dietary fibre naturally present in food," *Gut* 1995; 36:825–830

Ludwig DS, "The Glycemic Index: Physiologic Mechanisms Relating to Obesity, Diabetes and Cardiovascular Disease," *J Am Med Assoc* 2002 May 8; 287(18): 2414–23

Morris KL and Zemel MB, "Glycemic Index, Cardiovascular Disease and Obesity," *Nutrition Reviews* 1999; 57:9:273–276

Brand-Miller JC et al., "Glycemic index and obesity," *Am J Clin Nutr* 2002; 76(suppl): 281S–5S

McLaren DS, "Not Fade away — the Glycemic Index," *Nutrition* 2000, 16(2); 151–2

Morris KL and Zemel MB, "Glycemic Index, Cardiovascular Disease and Obesity," *Nutrition Reviews* 1999; 57:9:273–276

Wolever TM et al., "Comparison of regular and parboiled rices: explanation of discrepancies between reported glycemic responses to rice," *Nutr Res* 1986; 6:349–357

Ludwig DS, "Dietary Glycemic Index and Obesity," *J Nutr* 2000, 130(2S Suppl.) 280S–283S

Thorburn AW, "Slowly digested and absorbed carbohydrate in traditional bushfoods; a protective factor against diabetes?" *Am J Clin Nutr* 1987; 45:98–106

O'Dea K, "Marked improvement in carbohydrate and lipid metabolism in diabetic Australian Aborigines after temporary reversion to traditional lifestyle," *Diabetes* 1984; 33:596–603

Anderson JW and Gustaffson NJ, "Type 2 diabetes: current nutrition management concepts," *Geriatrics* 1986; 41:28–38

Fung TT et al., "Whole-grain intake and the risk of type 2 diabetes: a prospective study in men," *Am J Clin Nutr* 2002; 76:535–40

Bray GA et al., "Consumption of high-fructose corn syrup in beverages may play a role in the epidemic of obesity," *Am J Clin Nutr* 2004; 79:537–43

Rodin J et al., "Metabolic effects of fructose and glucose: implications for food intake," *Am J Clin Nutr* 1998; 47:683–689

Hansen BC, "The Metabolic Syndrome X," *Annals of the New York Academy of Sciences*, 1999; 892:1–24

Hsing AW et al., "Prostate cancer risk and serum levels of insulin and leptin: a population-based study," *J Nat Cancer Inst* 2001 May 16; 93(10): 783–789

Convit A et al., "Reduced glucose tolerance is associated with poor memory performance and hippocampal atrophy among normal elderly," *Proc Natl Acad Sci U S A*. 2003 Feb 18; 100(4):2019–22

Graham DJ et al., "Incidence of idiopathic acute liver failure and hospitalized liver injury in patients treated with troglitazone," *Am J Gastroenterol*, 2003 Jan; 98(1):175–9

Roberts SB, "High-glycemic index foods, hunger and obesity: is there a connection?" *Nutr Rev* 2000 Jun; 58(6): 163–9

Colcombe SJ et al., "Cardiovascular fitness, cortical plasticity, and aging," *Proc Natl Acad Sci U S A*. 2004 Mar 2; 101(9):3316–21

Steppan CM et al., "The hormone resistin links obesity to diabetes," *Nature* 2001 Jan 18; 409:307–12

Shuldiner AR et al., "Resistin, Obesity and Insulin Resistance – the Emerging Role of the Adipocyte as an Endocrine Organ," *N Engl J Med* 2001 Nov 1; 345(18): 1345–6

Styne DM, "Childhood and Adolescent Obesity," *Ped Clin N Amer* 2001 Aug; 48(4): 823–54

Eaton SB and Konner M, "Paleolithic Nutrition: A Consideration of Its Nature and Current Implications," *N Engl J Med* 1985, 312:5; 283–289

Ford ES et al., "Prevalence of the Metabolic Syndrome Among US Adults," *J Am Med Assoc* 2002 Jan 16; 287(3): 356–359

Chapter Six

Braunwald E et al., Eds., *Harrison's Principles of Internal Medicine*, 15th ed., McGraw Hill, 2001

Pennington JAT, *Bowes and Church's Food Values of Portions Commonly Used*, Lippincott Williams and Wilkins publ., Philadelphia, 1998

Lampe JW, "Spicing up a vegetarian diet: chemopreventive effects of phytochemicals," *Am J Clin Nutr* 2003 Sep; 78(3 Suppl):579S–583S

Weil A, *Eating Well for Optimum Health*, Alfred A. Knopf publ., New York, 2000, p. 108

Law M and Wald N, "Why heart disease mortality is low in France: the time lag explanation," *British Medical Journal* 1999 29 May; 318:1471–76

Shell ER, "The New World Syndrome," *The Atlantic Monthly*, vol. 287 no. 6, June 2001

DiMeglio DP and Mattes RD, "Liquid versus solid carbohydrate: effects on food intake and body weight," *Int J Obes* 2000; 24:794–800

Westerter-Platenga MS and Verwegen CRT, "The appetizing effect of an aperitif in overweight and normal-weight humans," *Am J Clin Nutr* 1999; 69:205–12

Williams MJ et al., "Impaired endothelial function following a meal rich in used cooking fat," *J Amer Coll Cardiol*, 1999; 33(4): 1050

Keys A, "Mediterranean diet and public health: personal reflections," *Am J Clin Nutr* 1995; 61(suppl): 1321S–23S

Chapter Seven

Hallfrisch J and Muller DC, "Does diet provide adequate amounts of calcium, iron magnesium and zinc in a well-educated, adult population?" *Experimental Gerontology* 1993; 28:473–483

Jancin B, "Many Physicians Already Reaping the Health Benefits of Antioxidants," *Pediatric News* May 1994

Fletcher RH and Fairfield KM, "Vitamins for Chronic Disease Prevention in Adults, Scientific Review," *J Am Med Assoc* 2002 June 19; 287(23): 3116–3126

Fletcher RH and Fairfield KM, "Vitamins for Chronic Disease Prevention in Adults, Clinical Applications," *J Am Med Assoc* 2002 June 19; 287(23): 3127–3129

"Nutrition Getting Short Shrift in Medical Schools," *Pediatric News* August 1991

Steele J, "Agriculture's Mixed Blessing," Ch. 10, in *The Third Chimpanzee*, 1992, Harper Perennial, New York

Eberhardt MV et al., "Antioxidant activity of fresh apples," *Nature* 2000 22 June; 405:903–4

Martin A et al., "Effect of fruits, vegetables, or vitamin-E-rich diet on vitamins E and C distribution in peripheral and brain tissues: implications for brain function," *J Gerontol A Biol Sci Med Sci* 2000 Mar; 55(3): B144–51

Abalan F, "Primer in Folic Acid: Folates and Neuropsychiatry," *Nutrition* 1999; 15(7/8): 595–597

Willett WC and Stampfer MJ, "What Vitamins Should I Be Taking, Doctor?" *N Engl J Med* 2001 Dec 20; 345(25): 1819–24

Wilcken DE and Wilcken B, "B Vitamins and Homocysteine in Cardiovascular Disease and Aging in Toward Prolongation of the Healthy Life Span," *Annals of the New York Academy of Sciences* 1998; 854:361–70

Kelley DS, "Modulation of Human Immune and Inflammatory Responses by Dietary Fatty Acids," *Nutrition* 2001; 17:669–673

Welch TR et al., "Vitamin D-deficient rickets: the reemergence of a once-conquered disease," *J Ped* 2000 Aug; 137(2): 143–145

Krebs-Smith SM et al., "Fruit and vegetable intakes of children and adolescents in the United States," *Arch Ped Adol Med* 1996 Jan; 150(1): 81–86

Benton D and Buts JP, "Vitamin/mineral supplementation and intelligence," *The Lancet* 1990 May 12; 335:1158–1160

Strauss RS, "Environmental tobacco smoke and serum vitamin C levels in children," *Pediatrics* 2001 Mar; 107(3): 540–2

Tannahill R, *Food in History* p. 45, 1988, Three Rivers Press, New York

Loraine JA, "Population, environment, medicine and global sustainability," *Ecol Dis* 1982;1(2–3): 167–175

Shambaugh GE Jr., "Zinc: the neglected nutrient," *Am J Otol* 1989 Mar; 10(2): 156–160

Kirschmann JD, *Nutrition Almanac*, Revised Ed., 1979, McGraw-Hill, publ., p. 230–31

Murphy SP et al., "Vitamin E intakes and sources in the United States," *Am J Clin Nutr* 1990; 52:361–7

Tangney CC, "Does Vitamin E Protect Against Cognitive Changes as We Age?" *Nutrition* 2001; 17(10):806–8

Sachek JM and Blumberg JP, "Role of Vitamin E and Oxidative Stress in Exercise," *Nutrition* 2001; 17(10): 809–14

Steinberg D, "Antioxidant Vitamins and Coronary Heart Disease," *N Engl J Med*, 1993 May 20, 328(20) 1487–89

Bove L et al., "A pilot study on the relation between cisplatin neuropathy and vitamin E," *J Exp Clin Cancer Res* 2001 Jun; 20(2): 277–280

Young IS and Woodside JV, "Antioxidants in health and disease," *J Clin Path* 2001; 54:176–186

Das UN, "Exploring the actions of vitamin C," *Canad Med Assoc J*, July 10, 2000; 165(1): 13–14

Kaufmann PA et al., "Coronary Heart Disease in Smokers: Vitamin C Restores Coronary Microcirculatory Function," *Circulation* 2000; 102:1233–38

Zitterman A, "Vitamin D in preventive medicine: are we ignoring the evidence?" *Brit J Nutr* 2003 May; 89(5):552–72

Bischoff-Ferrari HA et al., "Effect of Vitamin D on Falls: A Meta-Analysis," *J Am Med Assoc* 2004 Apr 28; 291(16): 1999–2006

Prabhala A et al., "Severe myopathy associated with vitamin D deficiency in western New York," *Arch Int Med* 2000 Apr 24;160(8):1199–1203

Raisz LG, "Homocysteine and Osteoporotic Fractures — Culprit or Bystander?" *N Engl J Med* 2004 May 13; 350(20):2089–90

Eaton SB and Nelson DA, "Calcium in evolutionary perspective," *Am J Clin Nutr* 1991; 54:281S–7S

Curhan GC, "Dietary calcium, dietary protein and kidney stone formation," *Miner Electrolyte Metab* 1997; 23(3–6): 261–4

Martini LA and Heilberg IP, "Stop Dietary Calcium Restriction in Kidney Stone-Forming Patients," *Nutr Rev* 2002; 60(7): 212–14

Zemel MB, "Regulation of Adiposity and Obesity Risk by Dietary Calcium: Mechanisms and Implications," *J Am Coll Nutr* 2002; 21(2): 146S–151S

Holt PR et al., "Comparison of calcium supplementation or low-fat dairy foods on epithelial cell proliferation and differentiation," *Nutr Cancer* 2001; 41(1–2): 150–5

Pignone M and Levin B, "Recent developments in colorectal cancer screening and prevention," *Am Fam Physician* 2002 Jul 15; 66(2): 297–302

Wu K et al., "Calcium intake and risk of colon cancer in women and men," *J Natl Cancer Inst* 2002 Mar 20; 94(6): 437–46

O'Keefe JH Jr and Harris WS, "From Inuit to Implementation: Omega-3 Fatty Acids Come of Age," *Mayo Clinic Proceedings* June 2000; 75:607–614

Connor WE, "Importance of n-3 fatty acids in health and disease," *Am J Clin Nutr* 2000; 71(suppl): 171S–5S

Marchioli R et al., "Early Protection Against Sudden Death by n-3 Polyunsaturated Fatty Acids after Myocardial Infarction; Time-Course Analysis of the Results of the Gruppo Italiano per lo Studio della Sopravivvenza nell'Infarto Miocardico (GISSI)-Prevenzione," *Circulation* 2002; 105: 1897–1903

Lands WE, "Eicosanoids and Health," in Lee KT et al., "Third International Conference on Nutrition in Cardio-Cerebral Diseases," *Annals of the New York Academy of Sciences*, 1993; v 676:46–59

Watkins BA et al., "Omega-3 Polyunsaturated Fatty Acids and Skeletal Health," *Exp Biol Med* 2001, Vol. 226(6): 485–497

Hibbeln JR, "Seafood consumption, the DHA content of mothers' milk and prevalence rates of postpartum depression: a cross-national, ecological analysis," *J Affect Disord* 2002 May; 69(1–3):15–29

Tucker KL, "Eat a Variety of Healthful Foods: Old Advice with New Support," *Nutrition Reviews*, 59(5):157–8

Cao G et al., "Increases in human plasma antioxidant capacity after consumption of controlled diets high in fruits and vegetables," *Am J Clin Nutr* 1998 Nov; 68(5): 1081–7

Christen S et al., "Gamma-tocopherol Traps Mutagenic Electrophiles Such as NO(X) and Complements Alpha-tocopherol: Physiological Implications," *Proceedings of the National Academy of Sciences* 1997; 94(7) 3217–22

Crocetti A and Guthrie H, *Eating behavior and associated nutrient quality of diets*, Anarem Systems Research Corp., New York

MRC Vitamin Study Research Group, "Folic acid and the prevention of neural tube defects: results of the Medical Council Vitamin Study," *Lancet* 1991; 338:131–7

Czeizel AE, "Primary prevention of neural tube defects and some other major congenital abnormalities: recommendations for the appropriate use of folic acid during pregnancy," *Paediatr Drugs* 2000 Nov-Dec; 2(6): 437–49

Russell RM, "Vitamin and Trace Mineral Deficiency and Excess" in Braunwald E et al., Eds., *Harrison's Principles of Internal Medicine*, 15th Edition, 2001, McGraw-Hill publ., New York

Haslem RH, "Myelomeningocoele" in Behrman RE et al., Eds., *Nelson Textbook of Pediatrics* 2001, 16th ed., WB Saunders Co., publ., Philadelphia

Tice JA et al., "Cost-Effectiveness of Vitamin Therapy to Lower Plasma Homocysteine Levels for the Prevention of Coronary Heart Disease," *J Am Med Assoc*, August 22/29, 2001, 286(8): 936–43

Sheiham A and Steele J, "Does the condition of the mouth and teeth affect the ability to eat certain foods, nutrient and dietary intake and nutritional status amongst older people?" *Public Health Nutr* 2001 Jun; 4(3): 797–803

McKay DL et al., "The effects of a multivitamin/mineral supplement on micronutrient status, antioxidant capacity and cytokine production in healthy older adults consuming a fortified diet," *J Am Coll Nutr* 2000 Oct; 19(5): 613–21

Bogden JD and Louria DB, "Aging and the Immune System: The Role of Micronutrient Nutrition," *Nutrition* 1999; 15(7/8) 593–94

Kuzniarz M et al., "Use of Vitamin Supplements and Cataract: The Blue Mountains Eye Study," *Am J Ophthalmol* 2001; 132:19–26

Lykkesfeldt J et al., "Ascorbate is depleted by smoking and repleted by moderate supplementation: a study in male smokers and nonsmokers with matched dietary antioxidant intakes," *Am J Clin Nutr* 2000; 71:530–6

Wooltorton E, "Bayer pulls cerivastatin (Baycol) from market," *CMAJ* 2001 Sep 4; 165(5): 632

Gaist D et al., "Are users of lipid-lowering drugs at increased risk of peripheral neuropathy?" *Eur J Clin Pharmacol* 2001 Mar; 56(12): 931–3

Fillmore CM et al., "Nutrition and dietary supplements," *Phys Med Rehabil Clin N Am* 1999 Aug; 10(3); 673–703

Cooper KH, *Antioxidant Revolution*, 1994, Thomas Nelson publ., Nashville

Bruce WR et al., "Possible mechanisms relating diet and risk of colon cancer," *Cancer Epidemiol Biomarkers Prev* 2000 Dec; 9(12): 1271–9

Langlois M, "Serum vitamin C concentration is low in peripheral arterial disease and is associated with inflammation and severity of atherosclerosis," *Circulation* 2001 Apr 10; 103(14): 1863–8

Harik-Khan RI et al., "Serum vitamin levels and the risk of asthma in children," *Am J Epidemiol* 2004 Feb 15; 159(4):351–7

Thomas MK et al., "Hypovitaminosis D in medical inpatients," *N Engl J Med* 1998 Mar 19; 338(12): 777–83

Holick MF, "Too little vitamin D in premenopausal women; why should we care?" *Am J Clin Nutr* 2002; 76:3–4

Gensini GF et al., "Classical risk factors and emerging elements in the risk profile for coronary artery disease," *Eur Heart J* 1998; suppl A: A53–A61

Guyton AC and Hall JE, *Textbook of Medical Physiology*, Tenth Edition, 2000, WB Saunders, New York, pages 900–901

Volpe SL et al., "The relationship between boron and magnesium status and bone mineral density in the human: a review," *Magnes Res* 1993 Sep; 6(3): 291–6

McGregor JA et al., "The Omega-3 Story: Nutritional Prevention of Preterm Birth and Other Adverse Pregnancy Outcomes," *Obstet Gynecol Surv* 2001; 56(5): S1–S13

Wood JD and Enser M, "Factors influencing fatty acids in meat and the role of antioxidants in improving meat quality," *Br J Nutr* 1997 Jul; 78 Animal feed: S49–S60

Braunwald E et al., Eds., *Harrison's Principles of Internal Medicine*, 15th Edition, 2001, McGraw-Hill publ., New York

Hoffman DR et al., "Impact of early dietary intake and blood lipid composition of long-chain polyunsaturated fatty acids on later visual development," *J Ped Gastroent and Nutr* Nov 2000; 31:540–553

Behrman R et al., Eds., *Nelson Textbook of Pediatrics*, 16th ed., 2001, Wm. Saunders publ., New York

Kruger MC et al., "Calcium, gamma-linolenic acid and eicosapentaenoic acid supplementation in senile osteoporosis," *Aging* (Milano) 1998 Oct; 10(5): 385–94

Chapter Eight

McGregor JA et al., "The Omega-3 Story: Nutritional Prevention of Preterm Birth and Other Adverse Pregnancy Outcomes," *Obstet Gynecol Surv* 2001; 56(5): S1–S13

O'Brien KO et al., "Calcium absorption is significantly higher in adolescents during pregnancy than in the early postpartum period," *Am J Clin Nutr* 2003 Dec; 78(6):1188–93

Wood JD and Enser M, "Factors influencing fatty acids in meat and the role of antioxidants in improving meat quality," *Br J Nutr* 1997 Jul; 78 Animal feed: S49–S60

Olsen SF and Secher NJ, "Low consumption of seafood in early pregnancy as a risk factor for preterm delivery: prospective cohort study," *Brit Med J* 2002 Feb 23; 324(7335):447

Kruger MC et al., "Calcium, gamma-linolenic acid and eicosapentaenoic acid supplementation in senile osteoporosis," *Aging* (Milano) 1998 Oct; 10(5): 385–94

Berenson GS et al., "Atherosclerosis of the Aorta and Coronary Arteries and Cardiovascular Risk Factors in Persons Aged 6 to 30 Years and Studied at Necropsy (The Bogalusa Heart Study)," *Am J Cardiol* 1992; 70:851–858

Allison DB et al., "Annual deaths attributable to obesity in the United States," *J Am Med Assoc,* 1999 Oct 27; 282(16): 1530–38

Giddens JB et al., "Pregnant adolescent and adult women have similarly low intakes of selected nutrients," *J Am Diet Assoc* 2000; 100(11): 1334–40

Johnson MA, "High Calcium Intake Blunts Pregnancy-Induced Increases in Maternal Blood Lead," *Nutr. Rev,* 2001 May; 59(5) 152–56

Simopoulos AP, "Genetic Variation and Nutrition," in *Evolutionary Aspects of Nutrition and Health: Diet, Exercise, Genetics and Chronic Disease,* Simopoulos AP, Ed., 1999, Karger, publ. Basel v 84; 118–140

Sue YS et al., "Decline in Physical Activity in Black Girls and White Girls During Adolescence," *N Engl J Med* 2002 Sep 5; 347(10): 709–15

Lloyd T et al., "Adolescent Caucasian mothers have reduced adult hip bone density," *Fertil Steril* 2002 Jan; 77(1): 136–40

Eaton SB and Nelson DA, "Calcium in evolutionary perspective," *Am J Clin Nutr* 1991; 54:281S–7S

Ilich JZ and Kerstetter JE, "Nutrition in Bone Health Revisited: A Story Beyond Calcium," *J Am Coll Nutr* 2000; 19(6): 715–737

Bottalico JN, "Diabetes in Pregnancy," *J Am Osteopathic Assoc*, 2001 Feb; 101(2): S10–S13

Galtier-Dereure F et al., "Obesity and pregnancy: complications and cost," *Am J Clin Nutr* 2000 May; 71(5 Suppl): 1242S–1248S

Connor WE et al., "Increased Docosahexaenoic Acid Levels in Human Newborn Infants by Administration of Sardines and Fish Oil during Pregnancy," *Lipids* 1996; 31 (Suppl) S-183–187

Davis MK, "Breastfeeding and Chronic Disease in Childhood and Adolescence," *Ped Clin N Am* 2001 Feb; 48(1): 125–41

Owen CG et al., "Infant Feeding and Blood Cholesterol: A Study in Adolescents and a Systematic Review," *Pediatrics* 2002 Sep; 110(3): 597–608

Stene LC et al., "Use of cod liver oil during pregnancy associated with lower risk of type 1 diabetes in the offspring," *Diabetologia* 2000; 43:1093–1098

Bennett M, "Vitamin B12 deficiency, infertility and recurrent fetal loss," *J Reprod Med* 2001 Mar; 46(3): 209–212

Zhang C et al., "Vitamin C and the risk of preeclampsia – results from dietary questionnaire and plasma assay," *Epidemiology* 2002 Jul; 13(4): 409–16

Botto LD et al., "Periconceptional Multivitamin Use and the Occurrence of Conotruncal Heart Defects: Results from a

Population-based, Case-control Study," *Pediatrics* 1996 Nov; 98(5): 911–916

Watkins ML and Botto LD, "Maternal Prepregnancy Weight and Congenital Heart Defects in the Offspring," *Epidemiology* 2001; 12:439–446

Rantakallio P and Koiranen M, "Neurologic Handicaps among Children Whose Mothers Smoked During Pregnancy," *Preventive Medicine* 1987; 16:597–606

Milberger S et al., "Further evidence of an association between maternal smoking during pregnancy and attention deficit hyperactivity disorder: findings from a high-risk sample of siblings," *J Clin Child Psychol* 1998 Oct; 27(3): 352–8

Yeo S and Davidge ST, "Possible beneficial effect of exercise, by reducing oxidative stress, on the incidence of preeclampsia," *J Womens Health Gend Based Med* 2001 Dec; 10(10): 983–9

Bennett PH, "Type 2 Diabetes among the Pima Indians of Arizona: An Epidemic Attributable to Environmental Change?" *Nutr Rev* 1999 May; 57(5):(II) S51–54

Hamosh M, "Bioactive factors in human milk," *Ped Clin N Am* 2001 Feb; 48(1): 69–86

Vik T, "Breastfeeding and cognitive development at age 1 and 5 years," *Arch Dis Child* 2001 Sept; 85(3): 183–188

Horwood LJ and Fergusson DM, "Breastfeeding and Later Cognitive and Academic Outcomes," *Pediatrics* 1998; 101(1) 99

Horwood LJ et al., "Breastmilk feeding and cognitive ability at 7–8 years," *Arch Dis Child Fetal Neonatal Ed* 2001 Jan; 84(1): F23–7

Mortensen EL et al., "The Association between Duration of Breastfeeding and Adult Intelligence," *J Am Med Assoc* 2002 May 8; 287(18): 2365–71

Birch EE et al., "A randomized controlled trial of early dietary supply of long-chain polyunsaturated fatty acids and mental development in term infants," *Dev Med and Child Neurol* 2000; 42:174–181

Bitman J et al., "Comparison of the lipid composition of breast-milk from mothers of term and preterm infants," *Am J Clin Nutr* 1983 Aug; 38(2): 300–12

Oddy WH et al., "Maternal asthma, infant feeding, and the risk of asthma in childhood," *J Allergy Clin Immunol* 2002 Jul; 110(1): 65–7

Williams GH, "Hypertensive Vascular Disease" in *Harrison's Principles of Internal Medicine,* 15th Ed., Braunwald E et al., Eds. 2000, p. 1414–1430, McGraw-Hill, New York, publ.

Singhal A et al., "Early nutrition in preterm infants and later blood pressure: two cohorts after randomized trials," *The Lancet* 2001 Feb 10; 357:413–419

"Propulsion and Mixing of Foods in the Alimentary Tract," Ch. 63 in Guyton AC and Hall JE, Eds., *Textbook of Medical Physiology*, Tenth Edition, 2000, WB Saunders publ.

Nicklas TA et al., "Family and Child-Care Provider Influences on Preschool Children's Fruit, Juice and Vegetable Consumption," *Nutr Rev* 2001 July; 59(7): 224–235

Wolfe WS and Campbell CC, "Food pattern, diet quality and related characteristics of school children in New York State," *J Am Diet Assoc* 1993; 93-1280–1284

Interagency Board for Nutrition Monitoring and Related Research. "Sources of calcium in the food supply" in Ervin B and Reed D, Eds., *Nutrition Monitoring in the United States. Chartbook I: Selected Findings From the National Nutrition Monitoring and Related Research Program*, Hyattsville MD; Public Health Service; 1993:89

Birch LL and Fisher JO, "Development of Eating Behaviors among Children and Adolescents," *Pediatrics* 1998; 101: 539–549

Carruth BR et al., "Prevalence of Picky Eaters among Infants and Their Caregivers' Decisions about Offering a New Food," *J Am Diet Assoc* 2004; 104:S57–S64

Hanson LA et al., "The immunological role of breastfeeding," *Ped Allergy Immunol* 2001; 12(Suppl 14) 13–19

Wold AE and Adlerberth I, "Breastfeeding and the intestinal microflora of the infant: implications for protection against infectious diseases," *Ped Clin N Am*, 2000 Feb; 48(1): 77–93

Sommerburg O et al., "Carotenoid supply in breastfed and formula-fed neonates," *Eur J Pediatr* 200 Jan-Feb; 159(1–2): 86–90

Reeds PJ et al., "Protein nutrition of the neonate," *Proc Nutr Soc* 2000 Feb; 59(1): 87–97

Picciano MF, "Nutrient Composition of Human Milk," *Ped Clin N Am* 2001 Feb; 48(1): 53–67

Schrezenmeir J and Jagla A, "Milk and diabetes," *J Am Coll Nutr* 2000 Apr; 19(2 Supp): 176S–190S

Taras HL et al., "Television's influence on children's diet and physical activity," *J Dev Behav Pediatr* 1989 Aug; 10(4): 176–180

Nicklas TA et al., "Family and Child-Care Provider Influences on Preschool Children's Fruit, Juice and Vegetable Consumption," *Nutr Rev* 2001 July; 59(7): 224–235

Troiano RP and Flegal KM, "Overweight Children and Adolescents: Description, Epidemiology and Demographics," *Pediatrics* 1998 March; 101(3): 497–504

Dietz WH, "Health Consequences of Obesity in Youth: Childhood Predictors of Adult Disease," *Pediatrics* 1998; 101:518–525

Roberts SB and Dalla GE, "The New Childhood Growth Charts," *Nutr Rev* 2001 February; 59(2): 31–36

Cavadini C et al., "US adolescent food intake trends from 1965 to 1996," *Arch Dis Child* 2000 Jul; 83(1): 18–24

Wildey MB et al., "Fat and sugar levels are high in snacks purchased from student stores in middle schools," *J Am Diet Assoc* 2000 Mar; 100(3): 319–322

Bittel J, "The Different Types of General Cold Adaptation in Man," *Int J Sports Med* 1992; 13:S172–S176

Ludwig DS et al., "Dietary Fiber, Weight Gain, and Cardiovascular Disease Risk Factors in Young Adults," *J Am Med Assoc* 1999 Oct 27; 282(16): 1539–1546

Young-Hyman D et al., "Evaluation of the insulin resistance syndrome in 5- to 10-year-old overweight/obese African-American children," *Diabetes Care* 2001 Aug; 24(8): 1359–64

Harnack L et al., "Soft drink consumption among US children and adolescents; Nutritional consequences," *J Am Diet Assoc* 1999; 99:436–441

Sweeney AT and Brown FM, "Gestational diabetes mellitus," *Clin Lab Med* 2001 Mar; 21(1): 173–192

Bottalico JN, "Diabetes in Pregnancy," *J Am Osteopathic Assoc,* 2001 Feb; 101(2): S10–S13

Stoll BJ and Kliegman RM, "Infants of Diabetic Mothers" in Behrman RE et al., Eds., *Nelson Textbook of Pediatrics,* 2000, 16th Ed., W. Saunders, New York

Aberg A et al., "Congenital malformations among infants whose mothers had gestational diabetes or preexisting diabetes," *Early Hum Dev* 2001 Mar; 61(2): 85–95

Morin KH, "Perinatal outcomes of obese women: a review of the literature," *J Obstet Gynecol Neonatal Nurs* 1998 Jul-Aug; 27(4): 431–40

DeGroot L, "High Maternal Body Weight and Pregnancy Outcome," *Nutr Rev* 1999 Feb; 57(2); 62–64

Galtier-Dereure F et al., "Obesity and pregnancy: complications and cost," *Am J Clin Nutr* 2000 May; 71(5 Suppl): 1242S–1248S

Elias SL and Innis SM, "Infant plasma trans, n-6, and n-3 fatty acids and conjugated linoleic acids are related to maternal fatty acids, length of gestation, and birth weight and length," *Am J Clin Nutr* 2001; 73:807–14

Allen KG and Harris MA, "The role of n-3 fatty acids in gestation and parturition," *Exp Biol Med* 2001 Jun; 226(6): 498–506

Black RE, "Micronutrients in pregnancy," *Br J Nutr* 2001 May; 85 Suppl 2:193–7

Bennett M, "Vitamin B12 deficiency, infertility and recurrent fetal loss," *J Reprod Med* 2001 Mar; 46(3): 209–212

Woods JR Jr. et al., "Vitamins C and E: Missing links in preventing preterm premature rupture of membranes?" *Am J Obstet Gynecol* 2001 Jul; 185(1): 5–10

Roth LK and Taylor HS, "Risks of smoking to reproductive health: Assessment of women's knowledge," *Am J Obstet Gynecol* 2001; 184:934–9

Zanardo V et al., "Labor pain effects in colostral milk beta-endorphin concentration of lactating mothers," *Biol Neonate* 2001 Feb; 79(2): 87–90

Hamosh M, "Bioactive factors in human milk," *Ped Clin N Am* 2000 Feb; 48(1): 69–86

Ulshen M, "Food Allergy (Food Hypersensitivity)," Chapter 338 in Behrman R et al., Eds., *Nelson Textbook of Pediatrics*, 2000, 16th ed., W Saunders, New York

Cunnane SC et al., "Breastfed Infants Achieve a Higher Rate of Brain and Whole Body Docosahexaenoate Accumulation Than Formula-Fed Infants Not Consuming Dietary Docosahexaenoate," *Lipids* 2000, Vol. 35, no. 1:105–111

Pan XL and Izumi T, "Variation of the ganglioside compositions of human milk, cow's milk and infant formulas," *Early Hum Dev* 2000 Jan; 57(1): 25–31

"The State of the World's Children, 1998: A UNICEF Report. Malnutrition: Causes, Consequences and Solutions," *Nutr Rev* 1998; 56(4): 115–123

Dietz WH, "Breastfeeding May Help Prevent Childhood Overweight," *J Am Med Assoc* 2001 May 16; 285(19): 2506–7

Jakobsson I et al., "Effectiveness of casein hydrolysate feedings in infants with colic," *Acta Paediatr* 2000; 89:18–21

Birch LL, "Effects of peer models' food choices and eating behaviors on preschoolers' food preferences," *Child Dev* 1980; 51:489–496

Rozin P and Schiller D, "The nature and acquisition of a preference for chili pepper by humans," *Motivation and Emotion* 1980; 2:77–101

Rozin P and Millman L, "Family environment, not heredity, accounts for resemblances in food preferences and attitudes: a twin study," *Appetite* 1987 Apr; 8(2): 125–134

Birch LL and Marlin DW, "I Don't Like It; I Never Tried It: Effects of Exposure on Two-Year-Old Children's Food Preferences," *Appetite: Journal for Intake Research* 1982; 3:353–360

Subar AF et al., "Dietary Sources of Nutrients among US Children, 1989–1991," *Pediatrics* 1998 October; 102(4): 913–923

Hyams JS et al., "Carbohydrate malabsorption following fruit juice ingestion in young children," *Pediatrics* 1988; 83:64–68

Interagency Board for Nutrition Monitoring and Related Research, "Sources of calcium in the food supply" in Ervin B and Reed D, Eds., *Nutrition Monitoring in the United States. Chartbook I: Selected Findings From the National Nutrition Monitoring and Related Research Program*, Hyattsville MD; Public Health Service; 1993:89

Petter LP et al., "Is water out of vogue? A survey of the drinking habits of 2-7 year olds," *Arch Dis Child* 1995 Feb; 72(2): 137–140

Robinson TN, "The epidemic of pediatric obesity," *West J Med* 2000; 173: 220–221

Must A et al., "Long-Term Morbidity and Mortality of Overweight Adolescents: A Follow-up of the Harvard Growth Study of 1922 to 1935," *N Eng J Med* 1992 Nov 5; 327(19): 1350–1355

Andersen RE et al., "Relationship of Physical Activity and Television Watching with Body Weight and Level of Fatness among Children," *J Am Med Assoc* 1998 March 25; 279(12): 938–942

Robinson TM, "Television Viewing and Childhood Obesity," *Ped Clin N Am* 2001 August; 48(4): 1017–24

Gortmaker SL et al., "Social and Economic Consequences of Overweight in Adolescence and Young Adulthood," *N Engl J Med* 1993 Sept 30; 329(14): 1008–1012

Venkat Narayan KM et al., "Lifetime Risk for Diabetes Mellitus in the United States," *J Am Med Assoc* 2003 Oct 8; 290(14): 1884–1890

Fisher JE and Birch LL, "Parents' restrictive feeding practices are associated with young girls' negative self-examination of eating," *J Am Dietetic Assoc* 2000; 100:1341–1346

Wildey MB et al., "Fat and sugar levels are high in snacks purchased from student stores in middle schools," *J Am Diet Assoc* 2000 Mar; 100(3): 319–322

Sallis JF, "Epidemiology of physical activity and fitness in children and adolescents," *Crit Rev Food Sci Nutr* 1993; 33(4–5): 403–408

Kohl HW and Hobbs KE, "Development of Physical Activity Behaviors among Children and Adolescents," *Pediatrics* 1998; 101:549–554

Moore LL et al., "Influence of parents' physical activity levels on activity levels of young children," *J Ped* 1991; 118:215–219

Pirke KM et al., "Early Pubertal Development and Overweight in Girls," *Ann N Y Acad Sciences* 1999; 892:327–329

Rocchini AP, "Childhood Obesity and a Diabetes Epidemic," *N Engl J Med* 2002 Mar 14; 346(11): 854–55

Chapter Nine

Kochanek KD et al., "Deaths: Preliminary Data for 1999," *National Vital Statistics Reports* 2001 June 26; 49(3): 1–6

Blair SN et al., "Influences of Cardiorespiratory Fitness and Other Precursors on Cardiovascular Disease and All-Cause Mortality in Men and Women," *J Am Med Assoc.* 1996 July 17; 276(3): 205–210

Mathers CD, "Gain in health expectancy from the elimination of diseases among older people," *Disabil Rehabil* 1999 May-Jun; 21(5–6): 211–21

Hu FB et al., "Physical activity and risk for cardiovascular events in diabetic women," *Ann Intern Med* 2001 Jan 16; 134: 96–106

Thune I et al., "Physical activity and the risk of breast cancer," *N Engl J Med* 1997; 336(18): 1269–1275

Ferro-Luzzi A and Branca F, "Mediterranean diet, Italian-style: prototype of a healthy diet," *Am J Clin Nutr* 1995; 61(suppl): 1338S–45S

Nestle M, "Mediterranean diets: historical and research overview," *Am J Clin Nutr* 1995; 61(suppl): 1313S–20S

Simopoulos AP, "The traditional diet of Greece and cancer," *Eur J Cancer Prev* 2004 Jun; 13(3):219–230

Bingham S, "Diet and colorectal cancer prevention," *Biochem Soc Trans* 2000 Feb; 28(2): 12–26

Blacklock CJ et al., "Salicylic acid in the serum of subjects not taking aspirin. Comparison of salicylic acid concentrations in the serum of vegetarians, non-vegetarians, and patients taking low dose aspirin," *J Clin Pathol* 2001 Jul; 54(7): 553–5

Anderson KE et al., "Association between non-steroidal anti-inflammatory drug use and the incidence of pancreatic cancer," *J Nat Cancer Inst* 2002 Aug 7; 94(15): 1168–71

Joshipura KJ et al., "Fruit and Vegetable Intake in Relation to Risk of Ischemic Stroke," *J Am Med Assoc* 1999 Oct 6; 282(13): 1233–1239

Garn SM, "From the Miocene to Olestra: A historical perspective on fat consumption," *J Am Dietetic Assoc* 1997 July; 97(7Suppl): S54–S57

Diamond J, *The Third Chimpanzee* 1993, Harper Perennial, publ., New York

Weisburger JH, "Eat to Live, Not Live to Eat," *Nutrition* 2000 Sep; 16(9): 767–73

Knize MG et al., "Mutagenic activity and heterocyclic amine content of the human diet," *Princess Takamatsu Symp* 1995; 23:30–38

Maric RN and Cheng KK, "Meat Intake, Heterocyclic Amines, and Colon Cancer," *Am J Gastroenterol* 2000 Dec; 95(12): 3683–4

Seow A et al., "Fumes from meat cooking and lung cancer risk in Chinese women," *Cancer Epidemiol Biomarkers Prev* 2000 Nov; 9(11): 1215–21

Blundell JE and MacDiarmid JI, "Fat as a risk factor for overconsumption: Satiation, satiety and patterns of eating," *J Am Dietetic Assoc* 1997; 97(suppl): S63–S69

Davis S et al., "Night shift work, light at night, and risk of breast cancer," *J Natl Cancer Inst* 2001 Oct 17; 93(20): 1557–62

Audette R, *Neanderthin,* 1999, St. Martin's Press, publ., New York

Ellis JL and Campos-Outcalt D, "Cardiovascular disease risk factors in Native Americans: a literature review," *Am J Prev Med* 1994 Sep-Oct; 10(5): 295–307

Yaffe K et al., "A prospective study of physical activity and cognitive decline in elderly women: women who walk," *Arch Intern Med* 2001 Jul 23; 161(14): 1703–8

Cordain L et al., "Physical Activity, Energy Expenditure and Fitness: An Evolutionary Perspective," *Int. J Sports Med* 1998; 19: 328–335

Keys A, "Mediterranean diet and public health: personal reflections," *Am J Clin Nutr* 1995; 61(suppl): 1321S–3S

Willett WC et al., "Mediterranean diet pyramid: a cultural model for healthy eating," *Am J Clin Nutr* 1995; 61(suppl): 1402S–6S

Kushi LH et al., "Health implications of Mediterranean diets in light of contemporary knowledge. 1. Plant foods and dairy products," *Am J Clin Nutr* 1995;61(suppl): 1407S–15S

Esposito K and Giugliano D, "Mediterranean diet and prevention of coronary heart disease," *J Endocrinol Invest* 2002; 25:296–99

Curtis BM and O'Keefe JH, "Understanding the Mediterranean diet; Could this be the new "gold standard" for heart disease prevention?" *Postgrad Med* 2002 Aug; 112(2): 35–44

Lorgeril M et al., "Mediterranean diet and the French paradox: Two distinct biogeographic concepts for one consolidated scientific theory on the role of nutrition in coronary heart disease," *Cardiovasc Res* 2002; 54:503–15

Cao G et al., "Increases in human antioxidant capacity after consumption of controlled diets high in fruits and vegetables," *Am J Clin Nutr* 1998; 68:1081–87

Alarcon de la Lastra C et al., "Mediterranean diet and health: biological importance of olive oil," *Curr Pharm Des* 2001 Jul; 7(10): 933–50

Fernandez-Jarne E et al., "Risk of first non-fatal myocardial infarction negatively associated with olive-oil consumption: a case-control study in Spain," *Int J Epidemiol* 2002; 31:474–80

Perez-Jimenez F et al., "Protective effect of dietary mono-unsaturated fat on arteriosclerosis: beyond cholesterol," *Atherosclerosis* 2002; 163:385–98

Visioli F and Galli C, "Biological Properties of Olive Oil Phytochemicals," *Crit Rev Food Sci Nutr* 2002; 42(3): 209–21

Kushi LH et al., "Health implications of Mediterranean diets in light of contemporary knowledge. 1. Plant foods and dairy products," *Am J Clin Nutr* 1995; 61(suppl): 1407S–15S

Akisaka M et al., "Energy and Nutrient Intakes of Okinawan centenarians," *J Nutr Sci Vitaminol* (Tokyo) 1996 Jun; 42(3): 241–8

Anderson JW et al., "Whole grain foods and heart disease risk," *J Am Coll Nutr* 2000 Jun; 19(3Suppl): 291S–299S

Dixon JB et al., "Reduced plasma homocysteine in obese red wine consumers: a potential contributor to reduced cardiovascular risk status," *Eur J Clin Nutr* 2002 Jul; 56(7): 608–14

Van Velden DP et al., "The Cardioprotective Effect of Wine on Human Blood Chemistry," *Ann N Y Acad Sci* 2002; 957:337–40

Craig WJ, "Phytochemicals: Guardians of our health," *J Am Dietetic Assoc* 1997 Oct; 97(Suppl 2): S199–S204

Joshipura KJ et al., "The effect of fruit and vegetable intake on risk for coronary heart disease," *Ann Intern Med* 2001 Jun; 134(12): 1106–14

Sinha R et al., "Dietary intake of heterocyclic amines, meat-derived mutagenic activity, and risk of colorectal adenomas," *Cancer Epidemiol biomarkers Prev* 2001 May; 10(5): 559–62

Rao CV et al., "Chemopreventive effect of squalene on colon cancer," *Carcinogenesis* 1998; 19:287

Smith TJ, "Squalene: potential chemopreventive agent," *Expert Opin Investig Drugs* 2000 Aug; 9(8): 1841–8

Gussow JD, "Mediterranean diets: are they environmentally responsible?" *Am J Clin Nutr* 1995; 61(suppl): 1383S–1389S

Stark AH and Madar Z, "Olive oil as a functional food: epidemiology and nutritional approaches," *Nutr Rev* 2002 Jun; 60(6): 170–6

Sierksma A et al., "Effect of Moderate Alcohol Consumption on Plasma Dehydroepiandrosterone Sulfate, Testosterone, and Estradiol Levels in Middle-Aged Men and Postmenopausal Women: A Diet-Controlled Intervention Study," *Alcohol Clin Exp Res* 2004 May; 28(5):780–785

Kennedy E and Davis CA, "Dietary Guidelines 2000 – The opportunity and challenges for reaching the consumer," *J Am Dietetic Assoc* 2000 Dec; 100(12): 1462–65

Jenkins DJA et al., "Nibbling Versus Gorging: Metabolic Advantages of Increased Meal Frequency," *N Engl J Med* 1989 Oct 5; 321(14): 929–34

Cummings DE et al., "Plasma Ghrelin Levels After Diet-Induced Weight Loss or Gastric Bypass Surgery," *N Engl J Med* 2002 May 23; 346(21): 1623–30

Roberts SB, "High glycemic-index foods, hunger and obesity: is there a connection?" *Nutr Rev* 2000 Jun; 58(6): 163–9

Grundy SM, "Multifactorial causation of obesity: implications for prevention," *Am J Clin Nutr* 1998; 67(suppl): 563S–72S

Guyton AC and Hall JE, *Textbook of Medical Physiology,* Tenth Ed., 2000, W. B. Saunders Co. publ., New York

Rajaratnam SMW and Arendt J, "Health in a 24-h society," *Lancet* 2001 Sept 22; 358: 999–1005

Martins PJ et al., "Increased plasma homocysteine levels in shift working bus drivers," *Occup Environ Med* 2003 Sept; 60(9): 662–6

Holmback U et al., "Endocrine responses to nocturnal eating — possible implications for night work," *Eur J Nutr* 2003 Apr; 42(2):75–83

Appendix 1

Exercise equipment

- Equipment for beginners in resistance exercises is inexpensive. Cast dumbbells are available in weights from 1 to 30 pounds or more, but the lighter ones are adequate for almost everyone. A set of three pairs (1-lb, 3-lb, 5-lb) should cost no more than $30, including a rack on which to store them.
- Adjustable weights are ideal for the experienced and conditioned exerciser. Prices and quality vary widely. They require a dedicated space, since you will probably also want to use a weight bench.

> *Caution: If there are young children in the household, store free weights carefully. Toddlers may be seriously injured by a falling weight and older children can injure themselves if they use the equipment without supervision.*

- Elastic bands are an inexpensive substitute for weights. They are convenient for travelers, and for elderly exercisers. They are usually available in graded sets.
- Exercise machines for home use usually occupy considerable space. Both the complexity and cost have an

enormous range. The less expensive ones tend to have thin padding and can be uncomfortable at the higher weight settings. Less costly combination units provide only a limited range of exercises. That can lead to boredom.

Some writers suggest the use of cans of soup, bags of sugar, etc., for really inexpensive exercise equipment. I doubt that anyone who has written about them has actually used them for more than a few days.

- Treadmills and track simulators are popular where foul weather is a disincentive to walking or running outdoors. Know what your exercise goals are before you purchase a treadmill. Pulse monitors, Internet-interactive connections and calorie-counters are incentive-boosters for some people, and so might be worth the extra cost.
- Bicycles, stair-climbers, rowing machines, and skiing and skating simulators are available for every budget. They all provide real benefits for persons who are motivated and committed enough to use them.

Appendix 2

Resistance exercise routines

THESE EXERCISES ARE only a few among hundreds that have been described in fitness and body-building books for the past 70 years or so. I have chosen them for specific reasons.

- They are simple.
- They are safe when performed properly.
- For most of them you will use the larger muscle groups and thus involve more muscle mass. That will ultimately result in a higher metabolic rate and provide more glycogen storage.
- Light weights (up to 5 pounds) are all that is necessary, although most of these exercises can be performed using standard fitness center weight machines. Two ordinary chairs are a sufficient substitute for a weight bench when you use light weights.
- Every major muscle group is used in this routine.
- More than one muscle group is involved in most of these exercises.

These exercises are for the beginner, especially for the one who is exercising at home. Use only light weights. More complicated exercises and heavier weights will require a padded bench designed for such exercises. When you can easily do 10 or 12 repetitions very slowly using the 5-pound weight, you may want to invest in more equipment or join a fitness center.

Caution: Always warm up for 3 to 5 minutes before doing resistance exercise. Cold muscles fatigue quickly and have a low injury threshold.

For the first 2 or 3 days of exercise, do them with no weight at all. You are preparing your blood vessels, joints, ligaments and tendons for the weight to be added later.

Repeat each exercise 10 or 12 times, rest about one minute and repeat the set. Although most manuals suggest 3 sets, the third provides little extra benefit. Rest about one minute before moving on to the next exercise.

Do all the exercises slowly, and do not hold your breath. Exhale during the positive phase, and inhale during the negative phase.

Allow a minimum of 48 hours before exercising the same muscle group.

School-age children always require adult supervision when exercising and should avoid heavy lifting. Specifically, adolescent and younger children should not begin bodybuilding or competitive weightlifting until they have attained skeletal maturity.

Do shoulder exercises such as the dumbbell press with very light weights, even after you have become well conditioned. The rotator cuff, a complicated structure surrounding the shoulder joint, is made up of several muscles, tendons and ligaments. It doesn't take much to injure any of these elements.

Push-up

This requires no weights. Beginners can start by using the bent-knee technique with knees touching the floor and later progress to the more demanding version, keeping the knees straight.

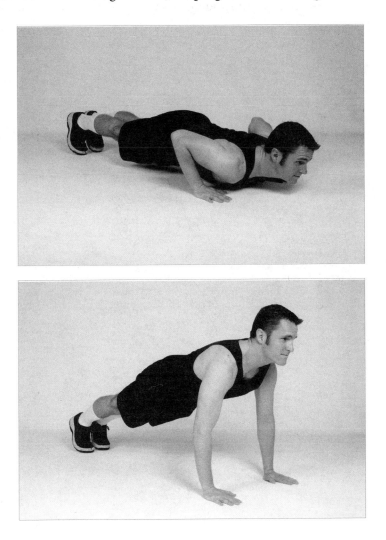

Seated overhead press

Start as shown in the first figure, with your feet flat on the floor. Push the dumbbells straight up, but do not lock your elbows. Lower them slowly to the starting position.

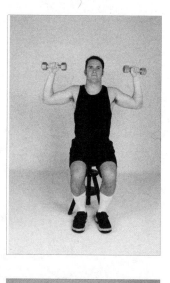

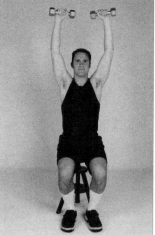

One-arm dumbbell row

If you don't have a bench, put two chairs side by side. From the starting position, looking straight ahead, raise the dumbbell straight up to your chest. Don't round your back or jerk the weight upward. Keep all movements smooth. Lower the weight to the starting position.

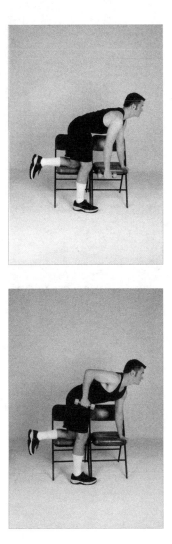

Triceps extension

Using the same bench or the two chairs, and the same starting position as the dumbbell row, straighten your arm and move the weight backward toward your feet. From this starting position, flex your elbow forward, then extend your elbow again.

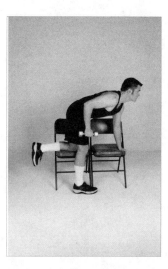

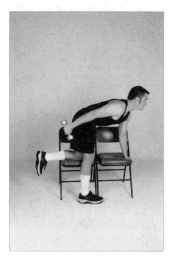

Hammer curl

Hold the dumbbells with your palms facing each other and your forearms parallel to the floor. Bending your elbows, curl the dumbbells toward your shoulders. Do not arch your back. Lower the weights to the starting position.

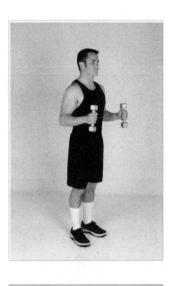

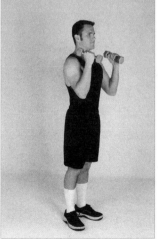

Half squat

Holding a dumbbell in each hand, with the feet about shoulder width apart, bend your knees while keeping your back straight. Your knees should form an angle no smaller than 45 degrees. Never do a deep squat unless you have no knee problems and are being supervised by a qualified trainer.

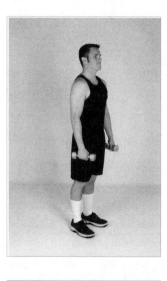

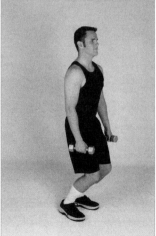

Stair step

With a dumbbell in each hand, step onto a stair using your right leg and then back down. Alternate feet and keep most of your weight on the stepping leg. Keep your back straight. I suggest that you do not use a stool for this exercise. We show it for illustration purposes only. A stair is more stable and safer.

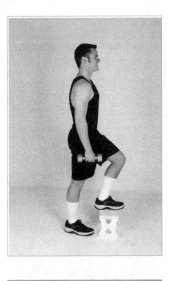

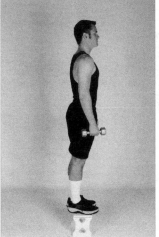

Abdominal crunch

Lie on your back with your knees bent and your feet flat on the floor. With your hands either behind your head or crossed on your chest, slowly raise your shoulders up from the floor a couple of inches. Lower your shoulders slowly. Do not hook your feet onto furniture or try to sit up completely. Do not push your head forward with your hands.

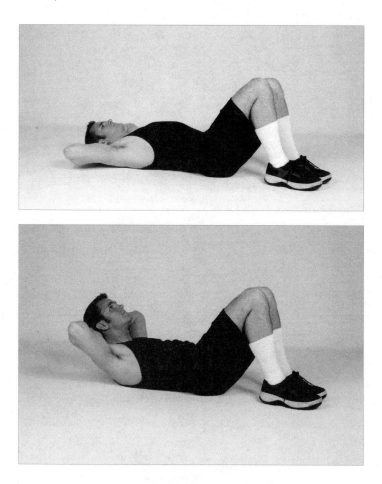

Appendix 3

Glycemic Index food rating

Suggestions for using the Glycemic Index

The Glycemic Index is a relative measurement; it is neither precise nor absolute. You will find values in other publications that may differ from these by 10 or 20 percent. Different brands of similar food products will vary by several percent. The listing below is based on the glucose standard, where glucose has a rating of 100 and white bread has a GI of 70. When white bread itself is used as a reference standard of 100, most foods will have a GI about 40 percent higher than they have using the glucose standard. The GI values listed below are based on the (lower) glucose standard.

Adding to the confusion of two different reference standards for Glycemic Index is the Glycemic Load. A food can have a high glycemic index, but you'd have to eat lots of it in order to raise your blood sugar. A good example is parsnips, which have a glycemic index of 97. However, there's so much water and fiber in a parsnip that you'd have to eat more than half a pound to reach the test range of 50 grams of carbohydrate. Only 3 ounces of Hershey's chocolate would do the same, and still leave you feeling hungry.

If you limit your intake only to low-GI foods you'll miss out on foods with excellent nutritional value (baked potato, parsnips) and pleasing flavor (honey, pretzels). On the other hand, not all low GI foods are healthy. For instance, chocolate has a GI of only 44, but not many nutritionists would call it health food. Other ingredients in a given dish or product (protein, fiber, fat, salt) will change the GI. When you shop for groceries, consider low GI foods as staples, and high GI foods as treats. Eating an excess of staples will make you fat; enjoying a few treats will not.

Low Glycemic Index — less than 55

Food	GI
Peanuts	14
Yogurt, nonfat, unsweetened	14
Soybeans	18
Cherries	22
Grapefruit	25
Milk, whole	27
Kidney beans	28
Sausage	28
Chickpeas, boiled	28
Yogurt, nonfat, fruit and sugar	28
Lentils	29
Butter beans	31
Apricots	31
Lima beans	32
Skim milk	32
Pear	33
Apple	38
Spaghetti	38
Fettucine	40
Apple juice	40
Meusli	40
Orange	42
Chocolate	44
Sponge cake	46
Carrots	47
Baked beans	48
Banana	51
Linguini	52
Sweet corn	54

Middle Glycemic Index — 55–70

Brown rice 55
Honey 55
New potato 57
Blueberry muffin 59
Sweet potato 61
Raisin bran 61
High fructose corn syrup 62
Ice cream 62
Rice, white .... 64 (wide variation: 41–104)
Couscous 65
Oatmeal, instant 65
Shredded wheat 67
Angel food cake 67
Sucrose (table sugar) 68
Rice, instant 68
White bread 70

High Glycemic Index — over 70

Watermelon 72
Mashed potatoes 74
Cream of wheat, instant 74
Puffed Wheat 74
Total cereal 76
Vanilla wafer 77
Crackers 78
Jelly beans 78
Pretzels 83
Baked potato 85
Potatoes, instant 85
Corn flakes 86
Rice Chex 89
French baguette 95
Parsnips 97
Dates, dried 103

Source: Foster-Powell K, Holt SHA and Brand-Miller J, International table of glycemic index and glycemic load values: 2002, American Journal of Clinical Nutrition, 2002; 76:5–56

Appendix 4

Reading references

The Paleolithic Prescription, Eaton SB, Shostak M and Konner M. Harper & Row 1987

Filled with fascinating insights, derives much information from modern hunter-gatherers about what life was like in the Old Stone Age. Available only in libraries.

Eating Well for Optimum Health, Weil A. Knopf 2000

Dr. Andrew Weil is a prolific author and lecturer with an unusual perspective in medicine. His botanical, cultural and pharmacologic interests combine to form a valuable bridge between traditional and alternative medicine. He is director of the Program in Integrative Medicine, University of Arizona School of Medicine.

Eat More, Weigh Less, Ornish D. Quill 2001

The lifestyle regimen that Dr. Dean Ornish recommends is a Spartan one, and not easy to maintain because it is primarily vegetarian and very low fat and emphasizes relaxation techniques. However, among the many writers on the subject of health and nutrition, he is one of very few who have validated their findings with peer-reviewed research.

Biomarkers, Evans W and Rosenberg I. Fireside 1991

Although the information in this book is more than 15 years old, it is not dated. The authors show conclusively that athletic ability declines only if we let it, and no one is too old to recapture much of the energy of past years with a sensible program of physical exercise and proper nutrition.

The Omega Diet, Simopoulos A and Robinson J. Harper Perennial 1999

Dr. Artemis Simopoulos has translated her experience and insight into a very readable presentation of omega-3 fatty acids, a deficiency of which is probably the most important nutritional error in the past half-century.

Nutrition Action Health Letter, Center for Science in the Public Interest

By subscription:
Ste 300, 1875 Connecticut Ave. NW
Washington DC 20009-5728

The Nutrition Action Health Letter is a burr under the saddle of business organizations and government bodies, but the positions they take on matters of nutrition have sound science behind them. Their recommendations regarding specific food items by brand name are easy to read and evaluate, and to put into practice.

Stretching, Anderson B. Shelter Publications, Inc. 2000

Eminently practical, this manual provides scores of stretching movements and exercises, and includes guidelines based on the sports activities that interest you most.

Those who complain about not having time to stretch or exercise will find helpful tips to eliminate that problem.

The Glucose Revolution. Brand-Miller J, Wolever T, Colagiuri S and Foster-Powell K. Marlowe and Company 1999

The authors have the ability to explain complicated science in an uncomplicated manner. The Glycemic Index is a swamp of seeming contradictions, but during a decade that has seen low carbohydrate diets cover the nutritional landscape, this team of scientists brings carbohydrates into the proper perspective.

The Essential Mediterranean, Jenkins NH. Harper Collins 2003

The term, *Mediterranean Food*, will never seem the same to you after you have read this excellent book. Nancy Harmon Jenkins gives colorful descriptions of the elements of the various Mediterranean diets and makes trying them easy with generously detailed recipes.

Index

About the author

PHILIP J. GOSCIENSKI, M.D. is a pediatric infectious diseases specialist with a 45-year career in clinical and academic medicine. He received his undergraduate degree from the University of Arizona, Tucson, and his medical degree from the New Jersey College of Medicine and Dentistry. Dr. Goscienski attained the rank of Captain in the United States Navy Medical Corps and was Clinical Professor of Pediatrics at the University of California at San Diego School of Medicine until his retirement from full-time practice in 1996. He continues to teach medical students on a volunteer basis in the Department of Community and Family Medicine.

He is a Diplomate of the American Board of Pediatrics and a Fellow of the American Academy of Pediatrics. Dr. Goscienski is the author of several medical journal articles and textbook chapters on various topics in pediatric infectious diseases. His articles have appeared in the *Saturday Evening Post* and other magazines.

His seminar program covers a wide range of health issues. For further information go to www.betterlifeseminars.com.

Dr. Goscienski is certified as a CPR instructor by both the American Red Cross and the American Heart Association. He is the medical director of a Public Access Defibrillation program in Oceanside, California where he resides with his wife, Patricia. He has five children and six grandchildren.